Keys to EMR Success

Selecting and Implementing an Electronic Medical Record

Ronald B. Sterling, CPA, MBA

GREENBRANCH PUBLISHING

Phoenix, Maryland

Keys to EMR Success: Selecting and Implementing an Electronic Medical Record

Copyright © 2008 by Greenbranch Publishing, LLC

ISBN 10: 0-9814738-1-4
ISBN 13: 978-0-9814738-1-9

Published by Greenbranch Publishing, LLC
PO Box 208
Phoenix, MD 21131
Phone: (800) 933-3711
Fax: (410) 329-1510
Email: info@greenbranch.com
Website: www.mpmnetwork.com, www.soundpractice.net

Requests for permission, information on our multi-copy pricing program, or other information should be addressed to the Permissions Department, Greenbranch Publishing, LLC. (800) 933-3711 or info@greenbranch.com

This publication is designed to provide general medical practice management information and is sold with the understanding that neither the author nor the publisher is engaged in rendering legal, accounting, ethical, or clinical advice. If legal, technological or other expert advice is required, the services of a competent professional person should be sought.

Screen shots of EMR products reprinted with permission from industry representatives.

Printed in the United States of America by United Book Press, Inc.

PUBLISHER
Nancy Collins

EDITORIAL ASSISTANT
Jennifer Weiss

BOOK DESIGNER
Laura Carter
Carter Publishing Studio

COVER DESIGNER
Jim Dodson

INDEX
Paul Hightower

TABLE OF CONTENTS

INTRODUCTION

The lack of effective medical record tools is dangerous for patients and intolerable for doctors and their practices. Without computerized support for patient services and practice operations, you must contend with inefficient operations and obstacles for doctors, staff, and even patients. In the final analysis, staff, doctors and patients are frustrated with the delays in patient service. Doctors and staff must sift through ever-growing mountains of paper to find the essential information and/or treatment plans for patients.

Unfortunately, few practices understand the challenges and demands of selecting and implementing an EMR. In too many cases, EMR decisions are made for the wrong reasons. In other cases, implementation is undertaken with too few resources and even less internal support. The result can be expensive ventures that leave members of the practice frustrated, maybe even angry.

Keys to EMR Success guides you through the demanding and challenging process of selecting and implementing an EMR. The book is filled with hundreds of tips, ideas, and advisories to help you avoid problems and achieve success.

From figuring out what you to need, to selecting an EMR and negotiating a contract, *Keys to EMR Success* will help you realistically focus on the key issues to consider and help you develop a balanced relationship with your vendor. After completing your contract, *Keys to EMR Success* will help you structure and manage implementation in a realistic and constructive manner. *Keys to EMR Success* presents strategies to preserve your EMR investment and insure that the EMR, and its use in your practice, evolves with your needs, and remains relevant to your colleagues.

There is no question that the selection and implementation of an EMR is a "bet-the-practice" proposition. If you fail, you end up with more costs and greater frustration. On the other hand, few practices will be able to avoid implementing EMRs as these tools become necessary to meet patient expectations, payer quality requirements and pay-for-performance demands. Understanding and accommodating the all-encompassing changes that EMRs produce will help you properly implement and effectively capitalize on these ultimately critical tools for your practice.

Properly implemented EMRs can provide a wide range of benefits to a practice and its patients. However, the implementation of an EMR is not an easy proposition. An EMR clearly demands a strategic vision and tactical focus. Attention to managing change and proactively working to keep the EMR relevant to your practice will help you more effectively serve patients and make better use of staff and doctors.

Keys to EMR Success: Selecting and Implementing an EMR was written by Ron Sterling, President, Sterling Solutions, Ltd., Silver Spring, Md. Ron, a nationally recognized expert, has guided a variety of primary care and specialty practices in over 30 states in the selection and implementation of electronic medical record and practice management systems. He has authored four books on practice-based computer tools. Mr. Sterling has reviewed electronic medical record and practice management systems from over 150 vendors. He can be reached via *info@sterling-solutions.com* or 301-681-4247.

AUTHOR'S NOTE

Doctors, medical practices and their patients suffer from the limitations of paper-based medical record systems and processes. Even with the best clinical and interpersonal skills, the limitations of paper records undermine effective interactions with patients. From taking a message instead of answering a question, to office visit delays in locating the expected test results (or even documenting if the test was done), patients are subjected to diversions from the quality of care provided by the vast majority of medical practices.

I have personally experienced practices losing requests for information about a family member in the hospital, and even the complete disappearance of a medical record with 20 years of information. I have waited for practices to find "missing charts," and witnessed doctor and staff frustration with the time needed to get their hands on important patient information. I have been given incorrect information on a medical situation, because the doctor could not effectively gather the complete information from the mass of paper that is my own medical record. Are these unusual situations? Am I the exception?

Based on my extensive work with doctors and staff in practices from 30 states, I know that the doctors, nurses and staff that serve patients are as frustrated, if not more frustrated, with the limitations of paper medical records. Fortunately, there are viable solutions to the problem. There are a number of practical EMR products, and the hardware prices have dropped. In the final analysis, practices need to value their own time and focus on improvements that can address the paper chase. Once your have achieved this conclusion, you must approach EMR selection and implementation with a serious commitment and clear understanding of the strategies and demands to assure success.

I would like to thank Beth Matosko for her help with the book.

Thank you,

Ron Sterling

Ron Sterling

ABOUT THE AUTHOR

 Ronald B. Sterling, CPA, MBA, President of Sterling Solutions, Ltd. (www.sterling-solutions.com), helps physician practices and other healthcare organizations capitalize on technology to improve patient service, clinical operations and financial results. Sterling Solutions provides project leadership and guidance to achieve tangible results and benefits from an EMR investment.

Ron is a nationally recognized expert on the selection and implementation of electronic medical record and practice management systems. He offers a full range of services to achieve success backed up by an extensive background in technology, physician practices and project management. He has reviewed software products from over 150 vendors.

With more than 30 years experience using technology and information as a competitive weapon, he has managed transitions to new computer tools for health care organizations in 30 states. He has served a wide range of primary care and specialty groups including some of the premier ambulatory organizations in the country.

Ron manages the transition to EMRs from conception to selection to implementation and deployment. He is vendor neutral, and focuses on the interests of the medical practice. He continually monitors product and vendor developments in this rapidly evolving and diverse software market.

He is a frequent speaker on EMRs to a variety of provider and industry groups including MGMA, TEPR, physician executive programs and Hospitals. He has contributed articles to a wide range of publications including *Medical Economics, and Ophthalmology Management*. He has also written "How to Select and Install Medical Practice Software" and the "Guide to Medical Practice Software."

Ron earned a B.S. in Information Systems from the University of Maryland and an MBA in International Business from George Washington University. He is a member of the AICPA and Maryland Association of CPAs.

ACKNOWLEDGMENTS

Writing *Keys to EMR Success* was actually cathartic and fun. *Keys to EMR Success* is based on real life EMR selection and implementation projects. The cathartic part was coming back from a particularly difficult situation and writing a book section about how to avoid and deal with the problem. The fun part was the open ended creativity that a book allows. Based on that origin, I am most thankful to the many practices that I have been privileged to serve and work with.

I would also like to thank Beth Matosko of Sterling Solutions for her help editing the book, and maintaining the list of EMR companies. Between mergers, and new products, as well as my obsession with certain aspects of the book, Beth has toughed it out with me in putting the book together.

Writing the book was one thing, but finding an appropriate channel and avenue for it is another. Maureen McCarthy, CPA of Snyder Cohn Collyer and Hamilton was kind enough to take a look at the book, and refer me to Nancy Collins of Greenbranch Publishing. Nancy and her team were enthusiastic about this book, improved the manuscript, and implemented their creative and comprehensive approach to publishing and distributing the book in your hand. The most amazing part was the speed and responsiveness that they demonstrated. Thank you to Greenbranch Publishing for freeing me up to work with my clients while they focus on the book.

Should I Invest in an EMR?

ven today, most medical practices don't have an electronic medical record (EMR.) And many practices that have an EMR have not generated the savings or efficiencies they expected. So, why should you make a major investment in an EMR?

Medical practices and physicians underutilize computer systems. Few, if any, other industries have so many key individuals going through their standard workday without any support or interaction with computers to support customer/client/patient service and their business purpose.

For example, car dealers and service stations have extensive recall campaigns for oil changes while the average medical practice does not have the tools to track or manage patient recalls for life threatening health issues. Some retailers are using radio frequency identification to track the location of a $50 case of paper goods, but medical practices cannot track the disposition of a battery of diagnostic tests costing hundreds of dollars. A service company can review every service call on your equipment for the past 5 years, but many practices cannot access a reliable list of prescriptions that the doctor has issued for the patient or quickly determine the pending immunizations for a child.

Physicians, clinicians and administrative employees are competing for access to and possession of the vital paper medical record. Without the paper medical record, the patient waits and the doctor is less efficient.

As you prepare to consider EMR, you need to contemplate the key differences between this effort and anything you have done. Before getting too caught up in the technological wonders of the EMR, let's take a reality check into the challenges that lie ahead:

Organizational—To take advantage of an EMR, your practice will need to re-think the way it works. From interactions with patients to the working relationship between the physicians and staff, the EMR will become a critical repository of historic and operational information that everyone will use. You need to re-design interactions with patients, other practices, payers and other outside parties. EMRs change the speed of information flow within the practice as well as the availability of information. Since the medical record is available immediately to any authorized user, the practice needs to determine the best processes to capitalize on and accommodate this dramatic change.

Management—Many EMR vendors like to portray system flexibility by offering that each doctor could use the EMR as he/she sees fit. In theory, your practice could pay several times to solve the same problem, and have to live with the consequences. The problems with inconsistent paper-based documentation do not go away with inconsistent EMR documentation. EMRs can offer a wide range of benefits to almost every practice but these benefits must be driven by practice policies that establish a structure to meet practice organization and patient care objectives. For example, each practice should carefully consider how their EMR is set up to insure that the collection of patient information will meet your care and documentation needs. Each practice needs to assure that patient information will be practically accessible to the wide array of doctors and staff involved in patient care. These strategies need the backing of the practice management team to insure that the EMR is used in a manner that most effectively helps the practice meet care and management objectives.

Procedure—EMRs will become an integral part of the practice's procedures and workflow. Indeed, you will have to account for the effect of the EMR on how you work as well as what every employee and doctor will do. EMRs will become the point of focus for every process and activity. Your practice will not be able to manage patient issues without the EMR, and you will have a vested interest in the ability of your staff to manage patient flow through the EMR. In essence, the EMR becomes the repository of patient information as well as the facilitator of patient movement, care items and messages. Practices that fail to recognize the pervasive effect of EMRs may fail to look for the correct features, and/or implement the EMR with fewer resources than required.

Technology—EMRs will dramatically increase the use of and reliance on computers for your practice and doctors. Arguably, you could walk over to your current practice management system (PMS), pull the plug out of the wall, and you will still see patients today. If you have an EMR, your tolerance for any disruptions will be limited since the lack of EMR access will prevent you from serving patients. You may go to great lengths to work around your current PMS because it may not be set up the way you want or need, or you may have outgrown the system. Unfortunately, you could end up in a bad situation working around the inadequacies of an EMR that is not effective. For example, you cannot view the outstanding orders for a patient, if the orders were dictated into a note that is stored in the EMR, but not entered into the patient order feature of the EMR. As important, you will need to invest money to mitigate the chance that you could lose access to your EMR. Practices may invest in redundant hardware and communication lines as well as extra workstations and tablets.

Staff—Most of the doctors and people in your practice do not rely on your current computer systems to do their job. With an EMR, everyone relies on the computers throughout their working day. As such, staff and doctors need adequate training, support on day-to-day use and a mechanism that insures that the EMR is available and relevant to patient care and practice operations. In some cases, this requires remedial training for staff and doctors who may have little experience using computers at all, let alone relying on computers for their activities throughout the day.

Regulatory—Due to increasing government interest in the healthcare industry, a variety of stakeholders are concerned that the government or some other regulatory body will establish standards or requirements that would make their EMR obsolete. Although the government has defined mechanisms to exchange information through the HIPAA transaction set, as well as standards for privacy and security, HIPAA did not require the replacement of existing systems in physician practices. Nonetheless, software vendors have added HIPAA features to their products to attract potential buyers. Using HIPAA as a guide, viable software vendors will add capabilities or modules to meet regulatory standards and remain competitive. That is not to say that all EMR products will have the resources to meet such challenges. Practices need to verify that their vendors have supported these requirements to date and are obligated to support future HIPAA requirements.

EMRs dramatically differ from the traditional use of computers in physician practices. Indeed, one would have to go back prior to the use of a computerized billing system to get a feel for the changes that lie ahead. EMRs are particularly challenging due to the following:

EMR Product Changes—Shifting from one EMR to another is much more complicated than making changes to your diagnostic equipment, PMS or other computer systems. EMR products significantly differ in how they track issues, store information and present patient charts. EMRs also differ in the support of clinical workflow. For example, some EMRs have special prescription refill management features. Buying an EMR to try it out, or buying a different EMR for various departments in the practice is a waste of your time and money. Ultimately, you could put your patients and practice in a risky situation. For example, having prescriptions on one software system, images on a second, and other patient information in a third could result in patients being given advice using less than all of the information that the practice may have. You should buy an EMR to achieve and support your patient service, operational and management objectives for the foreseeable future.

> ***TIP:*** Another important issue about EMR changes is the fact that you need to maintain the patient record for years. If you change EMRs, you may not be able to get all of the information that you need converted over to the new EMR and may have to maintain access to the old EMR for years after you finish using it. Therefore, pick the EMR that meets your needs and has the staying power as a product and company to avoid problems.

EMR Starting Point—Most practices have little to no existing computer-based clinical information and/or content to convert to the EMR. In most practices, clinical staff do not use computers to work with and serve patients. So you must formulate a variety of structures, strategies and procedures that are completely new to the practice. The practice needs access to the EMR from locations that may have no current workstations or equipment. For example, many practices have few computers in the clinical area since all of the patient information is in the paper chart. Additionally, most practices must train a number of users on how to integrate the EMR into their patient service style. Nurses will need to reference the EMR to know that patients are waiting for the doctor and/or the doctor has ordered a procedure or test.

Service Coverage—An EMR should support the variety of services, as well as support the workflow, between the clinical departments. These processes will facilitate patient services between departments, and support collaboration among doctors and staff. For example, doctors and nurses would issue lab orders to the internal lab through the EMR. The ability to call on staff and stay informed on patient issues instantaneously changes the working environment and time management of physicians and staff.

Strategic and Tactical Effect—The implementation of an EMR will have a dramatic effect on your practice and operations. An EMR will speed the flow of information in your practice, but you must redesign your practice to capitalize on these improvements. Many practices have failed to see results due to a lack of guidance and experience with these tools. To facilitate such a transformation, you need effective project leadership and management of the implementation process.

Looking at these significant challenges and effects, many practices have yet to pursue an EMR strategy.

EMRs AND THE HEALTHCARE INDUSTRY

Let's look at the healthcare industry and how you fit in. Today, you mostly exchange paper with a wide variety of players, including hospitals, insurers and other doctors. Typically, you send them your paper and they send you theirs.

Many practices work with healthcare organizations that have their own computers but produce few benefits for the practice. For example, some laboratories provide computer systems for practices to enter orders and print results that are placed in the patient's paper chart. Other organizations are providing onsite printers that print their reports at the practice. In other cases, hospitals provide workstations for physician order entry and printing of hospital information. In the final analysis, the practice may do the data entry for those organizations with computer systems, but these schemes produce few benefits for the practice. Indeed, the doctor may still need to record the orders, and, in some cases the results, in the patient paper chart.

This avalanche of paper includes a number of gems and important issues as well as a lot of "snow" that does not have a bearing on the patient's health and your business. Indeed, finding the important information in the paper blizzard consumes valuable doctor and staff time. In many practices, clinical staff "prepare charts" for patient visits by pulling important notes and pages to the front of the chart. At the end of the visit, someone must refile these pages in the appropriate place.

To get anything done, you have to co-locate the message or problem, the patient's medical chart and the doctor or clinician who will decide on the next steps. Typically co-location involves faxing information among your offices or passing charts around the office in search of the doctor. In fact, most of the faxing in many practices is to pass patient information among offices to get patient information to the doctor and/or, in some cases, maintain multiple charts for the same patient. In some cases, a staff person will read information to the doctor over the phone. In many cases, the issues must wait until the doctor has time to work through the stack of patient files on his desk. To serve patients, the doctor must wade through a variety of pages and notes to find important information. Doctors may note information or use dictation to record the patient visit.

Looking forward, the employer and government buyers of healthcare services are keenly interested in producing industry wide efficiencies through EMRs and the electronic exchange of information among healthcare organizations. Rising health care costs and an aging population fuel this interest.

Payers, and healthcare organizations that you do business with, want to eliminate the cost and inefficiency of paper charts and paper exchanges with electronic solutions. Whether a key payer starts requiring electronic information or patients come to expect a more timely response to their questions and problems, EMRs will become a required tool for physician practices to meet patient expectations and work with payers and other providers. In short, you may not have a choice whether to invest in an EMR.

Current industry issues that may affect your EMR thinking include:

Pay for Performance—A number of insurance carriers and Medicare/Medicaid are looking into pay for performance options that tie some compensation to support for quality measures. Quality measures can range from use of clinical treatment protocols to proactive management of patient care.

Medicare's 2008 Physician Quality Reporting Initiative (PQRI) includes 119 quality measures that are reported through the standard claims submission process. 2006 PQRI had less than 20 measures, while over 70 measures were included in 2007 PQRI. One of the more interesting aspects of the PQRI standard is that the reporting mechanism may cover a look back period for the condition. Included in the current PQRI measures are some quality measures that report on up to a 12 month look back window. Medicare is offering 1.5% of total allowed charges as a financial incentive. Regardless of your view of PQRI, an increase in measures as well as incentives (both financial and perception) is not beyond the realm of possibility. Keeping track of and reporting on these measures is difficult at least without an EMR. For example, the current coping "tools" consist of papers that are used to record the quality measures. But paper reporting tools do not help your practice determine if reports were submitted for appropriate patients, and how your practice is performing. More insurance companies could follow Medicare PQRI strategies.

Highmark BCBS in Pennsylvania awards pay for performance points for practices that have implemented an EMR (See page 7–6-43 at https://www.highmark.com/health/manual/Chp7-Unit6-1-06.pdf.) Many physicians expect additional pay for performance items that are based on having an EMR. For example, verifying clinical protocols, or following patient treatment plans are not practical without an EMR.

EMRs can help practices monitor compliance with practice level and industry level protocols while insuring that all doctors and staff can easily access patient care issues and outstanding treatment orders. For example, an EMR can identify outstanding patient care issues and orders for a particular patient when you access the patient medical record as well as in response to a general query for overdue services. Similar analysis of paper records would require an expensive and time consuming review of the paper charts for all patients. Such a review is not practical for many practices.

Common Care Standards—Medicare focuses on "prevention and early detection" and may raise patient expectations of care management and risk tracking. Your practice will want to be able to capitalize on such initiatives to improve patient service and management. For example, an EMR could help identify at-risk patients who have not been in for follow-up visits. Incidental patient contacts could be used to check up on patient compliance with clinical pathways and treatment standards. Examples of common care standards include

> **Bright Futures**—A health care standard for children from birth through the age of 21 (available at http://brightfutures.aap.org/web/) and

> **Bridges to Excellence**—Establishes strategies to improve care for targeted diseases (available at http://www.bridgestoexcellence.org/bte/)

Disease Management Initiatives—Many payers are interested in improving the management of patients based on clinical standards and guidelines. An EMR can support better management of patients with continuing care requirements and issues. For example, future services and testing can be entered and tracked as pending orders in some EMRs. EMRs can also present typical treatment orders for patients based on a particular problem or condition. Practices that can support disease management initiatives have more to offer patients, employers and payers.

Electronic Interfaces—The ability to exchange information among health care organizations is a key objective of the healthcare industry. Current electronic exchanges of claim and payment information between payers and practices are a small fraction of the exchanges that are done with paper. Additional electronic transactions will insure that healthcare organizations are better informed about patient issues through electronic exchanges including:

> The HIPAA Transaction Set (CMS Transactions and Code Sets Regulations, available at http://www.cms.hhs.gov/TransactionCodeSetsStands/) includes a transaction that allows providers to request specific patient information (Ex. Office Note, Blood Pressure) as well as a transaction that electronically returns the requested data. An electronic transaction that supports a full set of exchanges with pharmacies is included in the HIPAA Transaction Set.

> The Continuity of Care ("CCR") record supports sending patient information to a referred provider from a provider that is currently treating the patient. The Continuity of Care Record is available at http://www.centerforhit.org/PreBuilt/chit_ccrnyc.pdf

These transactions will allow practices and other healthcare organizations to more effectively collaborate on patient care and services. Providers without an EMR will not be able to capitalize on these exchanges and the resulting efficiency for the healthcare system as well as the practice.

Given that the healthcare industry is seeking to implement these changes, your practice faces a decision: you can establish a practice-based infrastructure to support these exchanges or you can print paper copies of information received and enter information from your paper records into a tool that will formulate the electronic transaction instead of an EMR. EMRs help you take advantage of the vast amount of clinical information that you collect but cannot practically access in a paper medical record.

EMRs AND YOUR PRACTICE

The reality for many practices is that an EMR will become an operational necessity and a cost of doing business in the next few years. Computers have dramatically increased efficiency and changed every other industry, and now the focus is moving to your practice. Nonetheless, you need to consider the specific needs of your practice including:

Size—Many physicians are frustrated with the lack of economies of scale as the practice grows. Expecting to see a variety of benefits from added size, many practices find that their existing procedures and policies do not produce a comparable benefit to the physicians or patients. A close look at these practices will reveal that many problems are caused by the larger number of people chasing after the paper medical record. Indeed, some employees will keep their own copies of various medical record documents to act as a back up. For example, many surgical schedulers, lab technicians, and triage nurses maintain a "shadow" patient record to keep track of their patient issues. In some cases, multi-office practices will keep duplicate charts for a single patient in order to serve the patient from multiple locations. Unfortunately, not all copies contain the same information. Working with outdated information can lead to problems. For example, a surgical scheduling form that does not have current payer information could lead to a rejected claim. In other situations, the cancellation of a procedure may be recorded on only one of the many different copies of the surgical scheduling form. Other employees and staff may not be aware of the change.

Quality of Service—In many cases, patient services and management are not provided as effectively and at the same level of quality as the clinical services. Patients may call in several times for information and are frequently put off until the practice can retrieve the medical record. With the paper chart, finding the appropriate information can take time. An EMR changes the patient service dynamic by providing instantaneous access to the patient medical chart and/or specific information in the chart. More importantly, the patient chart can be viewed in a variety of ways and the EMR can highlight important issues. For example, EMRs may allow you to view patient information by date of service, episode of care, or type of information (e.g., prescription list, outstanding orders). EMRs may flag pending orders and incomplete treatment plans.

Electronic Exchanges—To fully appreciate the current state of electronic exchanges of clinical information, let's look back to the early days of electronic claims. A number of insurance companies would actually give away PCs with their "key to disk" software that allowed your staff to enter the information into a computer and transmit the claim to the payer. The benefit to your practice was that the electronic claim was more quickly paid. The benefit to the payer was that you were doing their keypunching for them: the payers could eliminate rooms full of data-entry employees in the claims department.

Similarly, you may already be entering lab orders into the reference lab systems and reviewing the electronic results. Typically, the results are printed and moved around your office with other paper information. With the advent of clinical electronic transactions, you will be sending and receiving clinical information electronically. Lab interfaces are available with a number of EMR products. You enter and track tests on your EMR and results are loaded into your EMR. You may be able to review results on a flow-sheet and graph lab tests over time. You will be able to exchange clinical information and information on patient care issues through evolving transaction standards. These exchanges will become as common as electronic claims and electronic credit card transactions.

This book helps you work through the selection and implementation of an EMR. Following your analysis of the business case for an EMR (Chapter 2—Evaluating an EMR Investment,) the book examines your current computer situation (Chapter 3—Your Practice Management System and an EMR).

Proceeding through the selection process, the book will review compiling an evaluation list (Chapter 4), selecting products to review (Chapter 5) and actually reviewing the EMR products (Chapter 6). The book covers compiling your findings and making a final decision (Chapter 7), as well as negotiating a workable agreement with your chosen EMR vendor (Chapter 8). Succeeding chapters cover your implementation effort (Chapter 9), and the activation of the EMR (Chapter 10). Your continuing support efforts are itemized in the last chapter.

NOT BUYING AN EMR

Some practices will choose to wait to implement an EMR for a variety of administrative, political, management and financial reasons. Nonetheless, such practices should consider the following strategies to facilitate the implementation of an EMR in the future:

Paper Chart Preparations—Scanning of paper charts into an EMR is a monumental task. Unfortunately, practices do not design their paper charts to be scanned. Preparing a paper record for scanning is a major barrier to activating an EMR and takes 5–30 minutes per paper chart. To prepare charts for a future EMR, you may evaluate your paper charts and undertake a chart cleanup/reorganization process. The cleanup process may focus on eliminating old paperwork, unnecessary documents and duplicate documents. You may also seek to group chart documents that will ease a future scanning process. For example, if you decide that you will scan the last two years' worth of documents when you move to an EMR, you may want to organize your charts to support this plan.

Diagnostic Equipment Interfaces—When the practice purchases new diagnostic equipment, make sure that the new equipment will support an interface with a future EMR. You should get information on how you can interface with an EMR and include an option to buy the interface, if necessary, in the future. You can look for HL7 (Health Level 7 is an industry standard that supports the electronic exchange of information among healthcare systems and other devices) interfaces as well as a list of EMRs that the diagnostic equipment is interfaced with. Note whether the interface includes the study order from the EMR as well as returning the results to the EMR. These interfaces may be included in your future EMR evaluation list.

Transcription Capture—The vast majority of practices fail to capitalize on their investment in transcription. Typically, practices maintain word-processing files with the transcription, but do not store the files in a protected environment or with information to facilitate future loading in an EMR. To support future conversion to an EMR, your transcription files should include only one report for one patient per file. Some practices place all notes for a day in the same word processing file. Most EMR vendors would not be able to accept such a file into their EMR. Your transcription files should be protected from changes and editing, and include sufficient identifying information for the patient. For example, the patient's name, date of birth, gender and account number should be in the same exact place in each transcription file.

PMS Features—Several PMS products include workflow tools that support administrative based to-do's, and, in some cases, an imaging or basic EMR capability. Basic EMR capabilities could include a patient note capability and messaging feature. If you have such a product, seriously consider implementing the features that will let you capture key electronic data in a controlled structure. Potential options include an imaging capability to store images needed by many staff members as well as maintaining transcription documents. For example, you may scan in copies of the patient insurance card, and referral paperwork. Using these capabilities may help your practice in the interim. However, you need to preserve the integrity of your complete medical record in the paper chart.

Technology Strategy—Your practice should insure that any additional investments in technology will support the implementation of a future EMR. For example, replacing your PMS should include an option to choose your future EMR. Some PMS vendors have exclusive relationships with an EMR that may not meet your needs. Similarly, you may want to insure that additional workstations and communication upgrades can be easily used or upgraded to accommodate a future EMR.

Deciding to put off the implementation of an EMR may be the best decision for your practice. However, you should position your practice to more easily segue to an EMR in the future.

Evaluating an EMR Investment

EMRs can produce cost and revenue benefits. However, the expected benefits are not realized by many practices. The main barriers to realizing economic benefits are:

Insufficient Investment—For the vast majority of practices, an EMR will be the largest technology expense and project ever undertaken. Indeed, the EMR investment will significantly exceed the investment in your PMS. The costs can be justified by the fact that the EMR will have to serve a larger number of employees, and the critical nature of the EMR. However, some practices establish an unrealistic cost expectation. In order to meet the budget, some practices cut EMR hardware, training, and support. For example, practices that buy too little hardware will not allow for access to the EMR by all clinical staff. In frustration, some staff may start printing, and saving information from the EMR to get their jobs done. Other practices do not invest in hardware that can sustain hardware failures on a cost-benefit basis. For example, "hot swap" redundant disk drives can help the practice avoid lost data in the event of a disk crash.

Buying the Wrong Product—EMRs can vary widely in capabilities and features. Some EMR vendors will state that their product is not designed to support a paperless office, while other vendors offer their EMR by module. In the final analysis, your practice should prepare to fully implement an EMR to avoid paying for both EMR and paper charts. Otherwise, you may be better off not pursuing an EMR strategy. Some practices purchase the wrong product. The product may lack sophistication, clinical content (Ex. Charting tools for your specialty or area of medicine) or sufficient stability to be practically used. Practices may be lured into buying the product with the expectation that the vendor will make enhancements, and changes to address product deficiencies. For example, one practice waited three years for promised enhancements to address problems that prevent clinical charting with the EMR. Unless you want to expend time and resources to support the development of the EMR, you should make sure the product substantially satisfies your needs today.

Implementing a Less Than Complete EMR—Other practices stop in the middle of an EMR implementation. For example, some practices have bought all of the equipment, but only use the EMR to post charges and print prescriptions. In many cases, they end up with many EMR costs, but few of the benefits. The implementation of an EMR is certainly a challenge, but ultimately, the EMR is a strategic move that must be carried through to completion. Otherwise, the practice can end up worst off. For example, some practices have patient information split between the EMR and the paper record. The split complicates patient service, creates discrepancies, and risks problems with the designated record set, a HIPAA requirement.

Failure to Change Processes—Some practices use an EMR within their original paper-based workflow. The implementation of an EMR changes the information velocity and accessibility. For example, continued dictation may prevent updating the EMR list of medications and prescriptions to ease refill management. Similarly, an EMR cannot highlight incomplete tests when the test orders are in the dictated note, and not in the EMR order module. Some practices go to a lot of effort to make the EMR look and act like the paper system. For example, one practice would print the patient's record stored in the EMR when the patient presented for service. The printing of the patient record created a line at the front desk and kept the doctors waiting for patients.

Failure to Deploy Sufficient Hardware—Some practices fail to invest the money in the hardware to fully support the EMR. The basic challenge is to allow the doctor, nurses and staff to get access to the EMR from where they would have been normally working with the paper chart. For example, a stationary workstation in an exam room may prevent the doctor from maintaining eye contact with the patient during the exam. In other cases, practices do not provide EMR access to all of the people involved in clinical services. To save money, some practices limit tablets to the doctors. For example, one practice had nurses record intake information on forms that were entered by the doctors on their tablets before the doctor could work with the patient. In the final analysis, an employee without access to the EMR is analogous to preventing an employee from looking for information in your current paper chart.

The failures of many EMR projects can be found in the original scope, and planning for the project. To avoid these problems, establish a realistic expectation of the hard and soft costs for an EMR. Then you've set a strategic mandate to see the EMR project through to completion. In the final analysis, the strategic mandate will allow the practice to balance between the benefits of an EMR and realistic costs.

DETERMINING THE BENEFITS

An EMR will produce a variety of benefits for the practice. Some of the benefits impact revenue; others expenses. A number of EMR benefits improve services and productivity, but may be difficult to quantify financially:

Support Patient Collaboration—If serving a patient involves a variety of staff, technicians, or mid-level providers, an EMR will enhance collaboration on patient services and issues. By providing immediate access to information in the chart as well as outstanding patient issues, practice staff and doctors will be able to make better use of their time and avoid interruptions to track missing information. For example, immediate access to patient information may allow doctors to defer certain types of services to nurses and clinical support staff. Immediate access to the patient record may allow doctors and staff to address incoming patient calls when the patient calls and not later when they gain access to the paper chart.

Improve Documentation—EMRs enable practices to produce documentation on a more timely and consistent basis. For example, instead of the nurse recording information on a piece of paper that the doctor will dictate into their note, the nurse enters information directly into the EMR: the doctor only has to enter the new information or findings. Optionally, some EMRs combine dictated notes with information entered by the doctor or staff. Charting at time of service produces documentation when the doctor signs the note. More consistent documentation is enabled through use of a common set of clinical documentation tools as well as retrospective analysis of documentation for previous visits. For example, some EMRs allow the user to cite forward information from previous visits. More consistent documentation mitigates the risk of a patient service error, and enables all doctors and staff to quickly locate the appropriate clinical information. For example, doctors and staff will not have to adjust to the documentation styles, level of detail and placement of information (e.g., prescriptions and outstanding orders) for each person in the practice.

Improve Access to Information—EMRs allow doctors and staff to instantaneously access patient records. EMRs improve access to medical records by allowing doctors and staff to review patient information through a number of views. EMR records can be organized by date of service, type of document (*examples*: note, prescription, order), doctor, diagnosis and other criteria. Key information can be separately reviewed. For example, the user can see a list of medications, allergies, procedures and visits.

As important, EMR users can dig down into related documents by merely selecting the criteria and looking at the associated documents. Immediate access to patient records can cut the time needed to serve a patient as well as allow for immediate servicing of patient issues. With paper records, action on patient issues must be deferred until the paper medical record, and issue can be presented to the doctor.

More effective access to information is a significant benefit that can dramatically affect efficiency and productivity. Thrashing through paper records consumes valuable time for all doctors and staff. Paper thrashing steals time in increments that are difficult to measure and track. For example, an extra 15 seconds needed to locate the last prescription in a pile of patient prescriptions is virtually eliminated with an EMR. Add to that multiple 5 to 45 second delays thrashing for other patient information during each patient visit or the time staff spends reorganizing the patient chart before and after every patient visit. Eliminating paper thrashing will have a significant effect on how doctors and staff spend their time as well as how the practice is perceived by the patient.

Improve Patient Services—Patient service is inhibited by the inherent limitations of the paper record. Only one person can practically use the paper record at a time, and several pages may have to be reviewed to locate the appropriate information. For example, the nurse needs to access the previous note and reconcile the doctor's plan with other received documents (Ex. Lab results, MRI studies) to verify whether the information needed to serve the patient is available.

Patient messages and notes are circulating in the practice, but staff cannot easily determine the status and resolution of particular issues. Indeed, frustrated patients may call several times for the same issue and generate several notes that need to be matched up with a single paper medical record. Online access to patient issues and to dos as well as the medical record empowers staff and doctors to more effectively and quickly respond to patient queries. EMRs clinical orders, patient issues, and pending procedures can be accessed and reviewed by managers to track patient service issues and avoid lapses in care. As important, management will know with certainty the status and disposition of the various patient issues that the practice must manage.

Eliminate Lost Files—In many practices, lost files cause frequent interruptions to the staff and patients. Indeed, some practices have designated staff members who do nothing but look for lost files. Other practices return all files every day to the medical records department or employ someone at night to record information on the current location of patient files in the medical office. EMRs eliminate lost files and the associated disruption to the patient service process. All patient files are accessible through the EMR.

Even though the service and productivity improvements are substantial, you need to have a high level of assurance that the economic benefits of the EMR will offset the costs. The key economic benefits usually are:

Transcription

Practices that use transcription can spend from $1,000 to $2,000 per month per provider. An EMR can eliminate transcription expense if the physician charts patient information at the time of service. Unlike transcription, EMR charting can occur as the physician is seeing a patient. The physician enters the information into the EMR throughout the encounter. At the end of the encounter, the documentation is completed and transcription is eliminated. For doctors that dictate during the day, charting at time of service may allow for more patients. For doctors that dictate at night, charting at time of service will produce lifestyle benefits.

Numerous physicians are wary of charting at the time of service due to the impact on patient interaction, navigating through the computer screens, and being unable to change the record after signoff. However, the key issue is charting at time of patient service is a massive change to their patient service style. If the results improve the ability of the physician and staff to serve patients, then the change to charting will be worth the cost.

If the practice chooses to not chart at the time of service then don't expect transcription savings at he practice level. In the final analysis, charting at time of service is a physician decision. Some physicians may choose to chart all patients at time of service while other doctors may decide to continue using dictation. In any case, prepare for an extended transition period for the doctors and the practice. In general, concerns with charting at time of service can be addressed through appropriate clinical content, effective training, responsive support and the ability to amend the medical record as needed.

Medical Records

Medical record expenses include the costs of the medical record staffs, folders and materials, storage, printing and space. Hidden medical record costs include interruptions and delays due to lost medical records or the difficulty of finding information. In multiple office practices, faxing medical record information to the doctor can be a disruptive and expensive process. Practices with several offices may use up to 80% of their faxing to send clinical documents to another office or the billing department. A major productivity problem with paper charts is that many practice employees and doctors are competing for access to the same medical record.

EMRs eliminate the actual medical record expenses and allow everyone instantaneous access to the patient medical record. However, the practice will still need EMR support staff as well as staff to manage the exchange of paper records with other healthcare organizations. The initial transition to the EMR may include a scanning effort that will keep the medical record staff and additional resources completely absorbed for several months after the EMR is activated. Due to the EMR transition costs, the actual EMR costs should not be expected to go down for 6 to 12 months depending on your patient service cycle.

After the initial transition period, medical record expenses may drop by up to 50%. EMR patient file folder and paper expenses will dramatically decrease. A significant number of dedicated paper medical record staff will no longer be needed to pull, file, prepare and update paper charts. However, these resources will be initially dedicated to the EMR transition. The remaining medical record expenses will be needed to support the EMR operations.

EMRs may not produce any cost savings in offices that do not have medical record employees. For example, a satellite or small office, where several employees split preparing and processing medical records, will not necessarily see a decrease in expenses. That is you will continue to need someone at the front desk to greet patients and answer the phones, even if you do not need them to work with your paper charts.

E&M Coding Levels

Many physicians code office visits at a lower level than the services provided. Physicians may adjust coding due to concerns with the documentation quality or the belief that down-coding protects the practice from other problems. Unfortunately, down-coding prevents the physician from being fairly compensated for the services provided.

Some EMR products address this problem by calculating the E&M code at the time of service based on physician and staff charting. As the physician enters patient information, the EMR tracks the level of service. In many cases the additional revenue from more accurate E&M coding can pay for the EMR as well as mitigate the risk of a coding compliance problem in the future. Note that some EMR products do not calculate the level of service based on the information entered but on the factors selected by the doctor. For example, the product may display a worksheet that accepts the complexity and other coding factors from the user to calculate the E&M code.

Revenue enhancement from improved coding will vary widely depending on the coding accuracy of the physician. In some cases, the practice will see no improvement. In other cases, physicians may see $3,000 or more in additional revenue per month per physician for the same patient services.

> *CAUTION:* Some EMR products correctly calculate the E&M code for primary care visits but not necessarily for specialty visits.

> *TIP:* To estimate the effect of improved E&M coding, produce a report of the E&M code distribution for all of the doctors in the practice. Based on analysis of current coding distributions from sources such as CMS and subspecialty groups, project the effect of a more accurate coding on revenue. Review current distributions to identify providers that are not using appropriate codes. For example, some providers may always use Level 2 codes when the patients may really have deserved Level 3 or Level 4 codes, which pay higher. Comparing the expected distribution with the current E&M coding pattern will produce an estimate of the marginal revenue potential. For example, a doctor with only level 3 codes compared with a more evenly distributed provider may indicate that a certain percentage of the current level 3 visits should be level 2s and level 4s.

By calculating the expected payment for the redistributed codes, you can calculate the potential marginal revenue.

Pay for Performance (P4P)

Pay for Performance programs cover a variety of issues and practices. For example, some pay for performance programs pay a certain amount of money to practices that have and use electronic prescriptions, and/or an EMR. Other pay for performance programs are based on managing patient care items that require patient management strategies that are only possible with an EMR. For example, monitoring diabetic patients or patients with a heart condition requires automated tools to track last patient visits and diagnostic tests as well as effectively insuring that the patient comes in for the next recommended visit. In the future, pay for performance programs could depend on your ability to quickly identify and contact at risk patients and promote the management of their care.

> *TIP:* Pay for Performance programs are a moving target that you need to monitor. For example, the pay for performance factor that requires electronic prescriptions could be enhanced to require periodic patient visits for selected drugs. Be sure that you understand the strategic implications of pay for performance for you practice.

> *TIP:* Medicare's Physician Quality Reporting Initiative (PQRI) includes over 100 Quality Measures. Individual practices choose the appropriate measures to report and track. PQRI Measures include reporting treatment activities, as well as reporting events over a look back period of up to 12 months. EMRs can help the practice determine if PQRI reporting was performed when required as well as help the provider find the relevant information for those measures with a look back period.

Charge Capture

Many practices miss charges due to communication and process errors. Several studies have shown many providers miss several charges per day. Practices may miss charges due to recording problems in the office, lack of coding knowledge, and quick add-ons to patient services. Indeed, many practices dedicate complex procedures and staffing resources to minimize lost charges. For example, some practices use nurses to review all charts for lost charges on a daily basis.

In an EMR, all services and doctor orders are entered in the clinical chart to record the order and establish the framework to track the order through completion. For example, you may be able to identify outstanding or overdue services. That order information notifies other departments (e.g., lab, radiology) of services and pending patients. At the end of the patient visit, the doctor is presented with the list of services that were ordered and can initiate the posting of the services for billing.

EMRs also provide powerful research tools for coding staff. Patient medical records can be accessed on demand to review the actual record, billed charge information from the EMR and clinical documents to verify specific coding issues. Immediate access to the patient record will improve productivity of coding staff and increase coding accuracy. With a paper chart, the billing office may need to send a request to the clinic and the clinical staff may copy the relevant materials for transmission to the billing office.

To estimate the potential marginal revenue, the practice could audit a sample of clinical records for a selected day to estimate the missing office charges. Project the missing charges for a year to calculate the estimated revenue from missing charges.

Volume

Although most doctors have more than enough to do already, selected physicians have seen more patients daily with an EMR. The increase in volume is due to making better use of office time, support staff and facilities as well as the particular working strategy of the physician.

Physicians may be able to save time by having immediate access to patient issues and medical records through the EMR. Immediate access to relevant EMR information eliminates the all too common interruptions to leaf through the medical chart throughout the visit to locate the last note, test information or historical patient care issues. Additional time may result from elimination of dictation and more effective handling of messages and patient issues.

In some practices, doctors perform record keeping and transcription during the workday. For example, some doctors spend up to one and a half hours each clinical day on transcription. Charting at the time of service freed up dictation time to see other patients. For doctors who dictate after hours, charting at time of service will improve their quality of life.

These benefits will be realized after a physician is using the EMR effectively. In some cases, physicians may take a few weeks and in other cases physician may need several months to use an EMR efficiently.

Improved Collections

EMRs can improve collections by allowing the insurance collectors more effective access to clinical documentation on patient services. Instantaneous access to charts and E&M coding documentation empowers the biller to succinctly present the key information to the payer. For example, in the course of discussing a collection issue with a payer, an employee could call-up the relevant office note, and fax the note to the payer—more effectively and efficiently providing supporting information for claims.

More effective access to supporting information will help your practice avoid or eliminate denied claims that are not appealed. Nationally, 15% of denied claims are not appealed.

In many cases, the practice has provided the service, but lacks the supporting documentation that can withstand the scrutiny of an insurance company or support the dispute.

The practice should see an improvement in collections and virtually eliminate late-claim filling.

The worksheet below organizes your estimated cost and benefits for the EMR:

TABLE 2.1

Cost Reduction and Revenue Benefits Worksheet	Strategy/ Rationale	Current Expense	Projected Expense	Projected Savings/ Revenue
Cost Reductions				
Transcription Costs	Eliminate transcription expense for doctors who chart at time of service.			
Medical Record	Eliminate medical chart folder costs through the EMR.			
	Eliminate medical chart paper and copying costs through the EMR. Costs may include additional copiers that would no longer be necessary with EMR.			
	Cut medical record staff by half due to elimination of chart movement. This benefit will be phased in 9 to 12 months after EMR Go Live.			
Revenue Benefits				
E&M Coding Improvement	Calculate expected marginal revenue from a more accurate E&M coding method.			
Pay for Performance	Some payers are now offering pay for performance incentives based on a variety of factors. Calculate the pay for performance revenues that require an EMR.			
Charge Capture	Extrapolate the total lost charges from the sample charge review survey.			
Volume	On a physician-by-physician basis, determine the additional time available to physicians with the charting at time of service. Project the change in number of patients and apply the average revenue per patient.			
Improved Collections	Calculate late submissions that lead to untimely filing over the past year.			
ANNUAL POTENTIAL BENEFIT				

The total potential benefit will be compared with the estimated EMR cost below.

DETERMINING THE HARD COSTS

To save you time and money, a working budget of the EMR cost should be established early on in your process. Of course, the exact cost will be subject to final negotiations, but a working budget should be set up as soon as possible. The working budget establishes a benchmark for the practice as well as a reference point for your return-on-investment (ROI). As important, the practice owners need to understand the EMR scope and financial commitment. *Beware*: Most practices significantly underestimate the cost of moving to an EMR.

The understated cost estimates are based on experience with practice management systems, vendor cost estimates and optimistic scenarios. Practice management comparisons are inaccurate since more people need EMR access than the PMS users. PMSs are used by administrative staff, but the EMR must be accessible to every single clinical staff member and doctor as well as a number of administrative users. As important, EMR use is intense throughout the workday; sharing workstations is not practical. For example, nursing staff may share a workstation to review the PMS schedule, but, with an EMR, each nurse may need to access a different patient chart at the same time. Similarly, the EMR's list of messages and to-dos may be specific to each nurse.

Practices also invest money on a cost-effective basis in equipment and services that will minimize the risk of EMR loss, but may not be highlighted by the EMR vendor. For example, you may invest in redundant main systems, and spare workstations to insure that you can continue to access your EMR even if a particular item is out of service. Some practices also maintain backup communication facilities with remote sites.

Vendor cost estimates frequently exclude key costs. Vendor software costs do not include training, support, hardware and other items. In some cases, vendors may not include system software costs which are needed to run their system, but is not included in their EMR software license cost. Optimistic scenarios are based on what the practice perceives as a reasonable cost. However, many of these estimates are based on historic computer expenditures which are low for healthcare in general and certainly not designed to handle a major change to the practice's technology base.

Initially, you should determine what you consider a cost of the EMR, and what is not considered a cost of the EMR. A variety of items may be required to move to the EMR but it is your decision to require a comparable ROI or consider this the cost of doing business. This determination is not an issue of semantics since some of these investments may be needed by the practice whether or not they go to an EMR:

> **Workstation Upgrades**—Practices that are using a character-based system with basic terminals or have old PC workstations will probably need to upgrade their current workstations. EMRs frequently require more computing power to support the imaging data and other EMR capabilities. Additionally, EMRs may necessitate more workstations due to the constant need for most staff to have access to the EMR. For example, a workstation may be needed at the nursing station.

In situations where a workstation may be shared by two or more check-in desk staff, the practice will need a separate workstation for each staff member.

Network Upgrades—Data moves between the workstation and the server over an internal communication network and/or phone/high-speed lines. Your current system probably does not require the line speed needed by EMRs. EMRs require additional line speed due to the use of imaging in the EMR as well as the initial scanning of the current paper medical records. Upgrades to the internal network speed may be needed. Communication lines to your remote facilities may need similar improvement. Ironically, a number of practices have seen their interoffice communication costs drop when moving to higher speed connections. For example, an old connection used for PMS workstations was upgraded to a faster connection for EMRs at one half the cost of the slower connection since the practice had never renegotiated the contract for the old connection.

PMS Upgrades—PMS upgrades may involve upgrading your current PMS to the latest version. This could mean installing a new PMS as well as the training and data conversion for it. In some cases, the new PMS version may require a new server and even new workstations. In other situations, practices may replace the PMS as part of the move to an EMR. PMS upgrades are clearly the cost of doing business for a medical practice. However, the cost of integrating the PMS with the EMR product could be considered an EMR cost.

Compiling an initial budget can be complex and frustrating. However, the purpose of creating an initial budget is to set expectations and avoid future problems. For example, a practice established a budget of $20,000 for a 4-doctor practice. Another practice of 10 doctors wanted to implement an EMR for under $100,000. Given that a tablet device costs $2,000 to $3,000 and an EMR user license costs $2,000 to $4,000, the 4-doctor practice was looking at a minimum of $16,000 for the doctor setups without any money for other staff hardware, training, EMR server and other EMR essentials. Similarly, the 10-doctor practice needed $45,000 to meet the basic needs of the doctors without allowing for any other EMR costs.

You can compile an initial budget based on three strategies: **Basic EMR Estimate**, **Quick EMR Working Budget** and/or **Comprehensive Working Budget**. All three budget strategies are based on a 5-year amortization of the original costs of the EMR. Note that all three methods may not correspond to any quotes you have received since the budget may include items not in the vendor quotes, and the vendor quotes may have items that are not in the budget. For example, the working budgets do not include PDA applications for the doctors. The current vendor quote may not include a server with selected redundancies to cut the risk of a failure that could limit or prevent access to your electronic medical records. (The tablet on the next page will help you calculate a Quick EMR Working Estimate).

The **Basic EMR Estimate** is a monthly EMR cost of $1,000 to $2,000 per provider per month or $12,000 to $24,000 per provider per year. Communication expenses, mid-level employees, locations and a wide range of other factors can significantly impact this estimate. The basic estimate is based on general costs for a tablet, licenses, a low level server, basic training, implementation fees, and other costs. You can validate that estimate by completing a more detailed working estimate.

The **Quick EMR Working Estimate** does not include the details in the Comprehensive Working Budget, but does present a reasonable estimate of the EMR costs for the small to mid-size practice. The Quick EMR Working Estimate bundles a number of items that are detailed in the Comprehensive Working Budget (pages 23 and 24).

The Comprehensive Working Budget details the various items needed to implement an EMR. At a minimum, the Comprehensive Working Budget allows you check that you have included the various components needed to activate your EMR. The estimated costs column in the Comprehensive Working Budget can vary based on additional factors. For example, a very large practice could invest over $100,000 in their EMR server. The Comprehensive Working Budget Worksheet is at the end of the chapter.

CONSIDERING SOFT COSTS

In addition to the hard costs, EMRs require the expenditure of time and effort that are hidden and/or difficult to quantify:

Initial Productivity Losses—Most physicians are concerned about dramatic losses in their productivity as well as increased staff time. The implementation of an EMR is a massive change, but the impact to productivity varies widely by physician. Some physicians report dramatic improvements after a few weeks while others never get up on the EMR. The key strategy to minimize losses is to insure that you have one or more physician champions who can lead the way and demonstrate the results and benefits of the EMR.

> *TIP:* Each physician should carefully phase in use of the EMR according to the particular nature of their practice and services. For example, a primary care physician should start out using the EMR to document a single patient with a selected condition (Ex. Upper Respiratory Infection) on a selected day. The physician can add additional URI patients in succeeding days and then add additional clinical conditions. Thereby, the doctor is not risking problems throughout the day and with every patient.

Provider Time to Start Medical Records—Any EMR will require physician time to support the initial startup effort. Physicians must validate the clinical content for the practice as well as train and start use of the EMR to serve patients. Physicians must review the clinical content, establish the vision of how the EMR should work in the practice, and support the initial efforts to "Go Live" with the EMR. One or more physicians must lead the way for the rest during the implementation effort. Note that delegating the responsibility solely to nurses and other clinical staff will not build the physician skills or support that will be needed to deploy and use the EMR in the practice.

TABLE 2.2

Quick EMR Working Budget	Quantity	Unit Cost	EMR Total	Comment
Servers				
EMR Application Server		$15,000–$50,000		1 per practice to run the EMR, but you should buy 2 if you want redundancy for the EMR Server.
Imaging Server		$10,000–$25,000		1 per practice but some EMRs store images in the EMR Application Server.
Large File System		$20,000–$100,000		Larger Practices may need a large storage device to improve performance and security.
Backup Hardware		$4,000–$25,000		1 per practice
FAX Facilities Equipment				
Multi-Line FAX Server		$4,000–$10,000		1 per practice
System Software		$250/device		For each workstation and tablet
Printers		$1,500/printer		To upgrade old printers
Scanners				
Front Desk Sets		$300–$600/scanner		1 for each front desk station To scan a few pages from patients at the front desk.
Production Scanner		$2,000–$6,000/ scanner		At least 1 per medical record location to support Medical Record Scanning
User Devices				
Workstations		$1,000–$2,000 per workstation		Staff that share PMS workstations or have no access today may need an individual workstation.
Tablets		$2,000–$3,500 per Tablet		One tablet per doctor, nurse and clinical staff person
Application Software				
Electronic Medical Record (EMR)		$2,500–$4,000 per user		1 license per doctor, nurse clinical staff and others who access the current paper record.
Imaging Software		$500–$1,000/user		1 license per user
Installation		10%–30% of hardware costs		Varies widely based on number of servers, current hardware and a variety of factors.

— Continued

Continued from previous page

Quick EMR Working Budget	Quantity	Unit Cost	EMR Total	Comment
Training		40% to 60% of EMR Application Costs		Varies widely based on training strategy, location, and staff sophistication.
TOTALS				
Hardware Contingency				Allows for unexpected upgrades to hardware.
Other Contingency				Covers other potential costs that are not covered elsewhere.
Services Contingency				Supports additional training and implementation services for practices with complex situations.
TOTAL WITH CONTINGENCY				

Staff Time to Start Medical Records—An EMR necessitates a complete change to the way the staff works and manages patient care. The change to workflow will require a significant amount of time to develop, and deploy the changes as well as train and support staff. The transition of patient paper charts to the EMR is a massive undertaking for any practice. Transition activities may include scanning paper charts, back loading information into the EMR from the charts and/or setting up an existing patient on their first EMR visit. For example, you may have to load in previous procedures into the EMR and existing problems to take advantage of the EMR Patient Summary Screen. The startup efforts will absorb all of your current staff time and then some from the time you select your EMR until at least 6 months after the EMR is activated.

Unexpected Upgrades to Current Computers and Communications—In many practices, some current workstations and communications must be upgraded to support the EMR. Additionally, current versions of key software may not be the most current version required by the EMR. For example, you may need to upgrade your practice management system, and purchase an interface for the EMR to exchange data with the PMS. The communications network designed for the PMS may not be sufficient for EMR volumes and images. Note that communications changes could affect intra-office and inter-office communications. For example, a slow router may require replacement to increase the speed of the network in the office, while a slow direct dial-up or DSL connection must be upgraded to a faster T1 connection.

> *TIP:* Unfortunately, these communications upgrades can have an extended lead time for installation and activation. For example, a new communication service between your office and a satellite may take 30 to 90 days to deploy. Make sure that you time you communications orders to avoid delays to the rest of the project.

Additional Security and Network Protection—EMRs significantly raise the security and network protection requirements for a practice. Internet access without controls, unprotected workstations and lax system security policies will cost a practice a lot of time, effort and money. For example, a practice had a serious problem with a software virus that was introduced from software that was loaded on their system by accident. The practice must evaluate security vulnerabilities and address those issues for the initial implementation as well as establish procedures to monitor security. For example, changing passwords on a periodic basis is an important security procedure.

Continuing Staff and Provider Support—The practice must establish a continuing process to support staff and manage changes to the EMR. Ad hoc changes to EMR standards and procedures expose the practice to a variety of risks and undermine the EMR investment.

> **TIP:** You should establish a continuing process to assure all users are properly trained in the use of the EMR as well as how the EMR is used at the practice. For example, a standard training and mentoring strategy for new clinical employees will help maintain the appropriate level of expertise and standards for the EMR.

The working EMR budget will go through several iterations as the project moves forward. The working budget format can be used to compare products, as well as manage the budget.

INVESTMENT ANALYSIS

After calculating the cost and the projected benefits, you can now analyze your EMR investment. In general, larger practices will develop a more compelling financial reason to implement an EMR. The relation between size and benefits is directly related to the number of people who access the paper chart. In smaller practices, the competition for patient information is not as fierce since patient service involves fewer people. If your practice has more than one person working on care for a particular patient, then your practice is well positioned to capitalize on an EMR. If your practice has been frustrated with the lack of economies of scale even as you have grown, then the EMR may help you generate these benefits.

But a financial return on EMRs will make the decision easier. The worksheet on page 26 helps you calculate a return on investment based on the information you gathered above. Note the worksheet spreads the initial costs (A) over a 5-year period.

Note that the EMR Return on Investment does not include interest expenses, soft costs or the phase-in of benefits noted above. However, the worksheet does present the magnitude of the project and potential benefits.

If the benefits and marginal revenues present a compelling return on your EMR investment, that is great. However, the lack of a compelling ROI may not necessarily free you from the business need to implement an EMR. You need to consider the competitive is-

TABLE 2.3

EMR Return on Investment	Amount	Comment
A. Cost Estimate		Cost estimate from one of the three strategies listed above.
B. Five Year Annualized Cost		Divide A. by 5 to calculate the annual cost over the first 5 years (For Basic EMR Estimate, multiply monthly cost by 12)
C. Annual EMR Software Support		Add Annual Software Support of 18% to 33% of the original software cost (0 for Basic EMR Estimate)
D. Annual EMR Hardware Support		Add Annual Hardware Support of 12% of the Hardware Cost (0 for Basic EMR Estimate)
Total Annual Costs		**Sum of B, C, and D.**
E. ANNUAL POTENTIAL BENEFIT		From Cost Reduction and Revenue Benefits Worksheet Above.
F. Annual Potential Profit or Loss on EMR Investment		Subtract Total Expected Costs (D) from Annual Potential Benefit (E)

sues, patient expectations and the general movement of the healthcare industry to insure that you maintain a responsive and viable practice. Otherwise, you may be left at a disadvantage. For example, practices that can interact with patients over the Internet provide an alternative to waiting on hold to schedule an appointment or request a refill.

TABLE 2.4

Comprehensive Working Budget	Item	Purpose	Key Issues	Estimated Costs
Hardware	EMR Server	EMR servers contain the medical record information and the EMR application. In most cases, the EMR operates on a different server than the PMS application.	Various levels of protection from server failure can be purchased. A cluster server includes two or more servers sharing the same data repository. Cluster servers can continue to provide service in the event of a serious problem with one of the servers in a cluster.	$15,000–$250,000
	Image Server	Many EMR products store images on a separate server. The server contains the images that are accessed through the EMR. EMRs that use a single server for both the EMR and imaging do not require a dedicated Image Server.	Image volume can be very substantial. Scanning of current paper records as well as storing new incoming documents and images may require very large storage capacity.	$10,000–$30,000
	Storage System	EMRs may store massive amounts of information and images. A Storage Area Network (SAN) allows you to accommodate large amounts of data and images in a fast and secure environment. Not all practices need a SAN.	Larger practices may need the SAN to handle the amount of information as well as provide a viable way to backup all of the data.	$20,000–$150,000
	Backup System	EMRs contain much more data than you collect with a PMS system. The backup system may be attached to one of the main servers (e.g., EMR Server).	A dedicated backup server may allow for greater flexibility by downloading the information to the backup server storage, and backing up the storage to tape. PMS backup devices are mostly too slow to handle EMR backups.	$4,000–$35,000
	Interface Server	In the event that your EMR will be interfacing with a PMS, PACS, or other systems, you may need an interface server. In some cases, EMRs exchange information without an interface server. Without an interface server, the information is sent as a transaction between the PMS and EMR.	The interface between the EMR and the PMS may conflict with each other and require additional equipment or testing.	$4,000–$10,000
	FAX Server	Incoming faxes will be immediately entered into the EMR in paperless environments. Otherwise, you would need to scan the fax into the EMR and store the image in the EMR. Fax servers accept the image of the Fax, and track incoming faxes. The fax server bypasses the print and scanning process to add the image to the EMR.	Many EMR vendors do not offer fax servers. An alternative to fax servers are Internet-based services that deliver your incoming fax as an email with an image attachment.	$5,000–$10,000

— Continued

Continued from previous page

Comprehensive Working Budget	Item	Purpose	Key Issues	Estimated Costs
	Other System Servers	To support a computer network, you may need additional servers to manage overhead issues. Overhead issues include email (Mail Server), printer management (Print Server), and network traffic management (Domain Server and Active Directory Server.)	If you currently have a network, you may still need to upgrade the additional servers for additional capacity, and/or backup the key servers.	$4,000–$8,000 per server.
	Remote Workstation Server	Remote workstation servers allow you to improve the support for wireless devices and decrease the communications needed for remote offices. Basically, remote workstation servers act as a local proxy for a remote user (like *PC Anywhere*). All of the information that is typically exchanged between the workstation and the EMR server is done locally in your computer room; only the screen information is transmitted to the remote user. The remote EMR uses fewer communication resources than without the remote workstation server. Some EMRs are based on technologies that eliminate the need for remote workstation servers. Note that ASPs typically provide the remote workstation facilities for practices using their service.	Remote servers also help mitigate lost data due to communication problems or interruptions in contact with the remote user. Remote workstation servers improve and simplify management of the system since you can affect many users through working with the remote workstation sever. Costs of Remote Workstation Servers can vary widely and is impacted by the number of users.	$10,000–$40,000.
	Network Infrastructure	A wireless network will be needed to support the EMR at each location. A variety of options exist. The wireless network should be considered with any other improvements to the communication infrastructure.	Locations may need multiple access points based on size, interference and other factors.	$700–$3,000 per location
System Software	Network Access Licenses	Workstations and Tablets on a network require licenses to access the servers. Licenses may also be needed to access applications, such as email.	A variety of network licenses may be needed including access, virus protection and other facilities. These requirements vary widely by vendor and can be impacted by your own installed systems. For example, you may need a special terminal emulation program to access the current PMS application from the new EMR workstations.	$40–$200 per workstations/ tablet.

— Continued

Continued from previous page

Comprehensive Working Budget	Item	Purpose	Key Issues	Estimated Costs
	Database Access Licenses	Most EMRs are built on a database system. Many database vendors require each user or each workstation/tablet to have a database license.	In some cases, the EMR vendors include the database license in the EMR costs.	$100–$250 per workstation/use
Tablets and Workstations	Additional Workstations	Additional workstations may be needed to support users who will need EMR access but do not have current access to a workstation. Additional users may be found in the clinical and administrative area. For example, procedure schedulers and insurance collectors will need access to the EMR. With workflow features, virtually every employee and doctor needs EMR access.	Workstations may be needed for staff who share workstations with other employees as well as staff who use the medical chart, but have no workstations today. Additional workstations may be allocated for nursing stations, doctor offices and other locations, as needed.	$1,000–$1,500 per workstation.
	Tablets	Virtually every doctor, nurse and clinical worker will need access to the EMR. If the person in question moves around to serve patients, he may need a tablet instead of a workstation. Tablets communicate with the EMR over radio frequency connections and allow the user to maintain contact with the system as they move around the facility. Tablets also simplify HIPAA Privacy and Security compliance. For example, if a workstation was in each exam room, the screen would have to be secured each time the user left the room.	The practice needs a strategy to accommodate doctors and staff who move between facilities. Tablets may be shared by part-time employees. Each location needs tablets for peak staffing. Each location may need a spare tablet.	$2,000–$3,500 per tablet.
Printers	Color Printers	Color printers can print patient education information from the EMR and other sources.	Some practices do not use color printers since they are more expensive and slower than other printers.	$500–$3,000 per printer
	Other Printers	Additional printers may be needed to support the EMR.	The practice may replace old PMS printers to improve print quality for EMR products.	$300–$2,500 per printer

Continued from previous page

Comprehensive Working Budget	Item	Purpose	Key Issues	Estimated Costs
Scanners	Front Desk Scanners	Front desks will receive miscellaneous forms, reports and information from presenting patients. Typically, the patient only has a few pages. Due to space constraints at most front desks, a small hand-fed scanner has been successful in a number of practices.	Small scanners may be needed by other staff that may receive a few pages from patients. Nurses and surgery schedulers may need small scanners.	$200–$600 per sheet-scanner.
	High Volume Scanners	To maintain the designated record set, some practices scan the existing paper records into the EMR. Scanning old paper charts requires a faster, heavy duty scanner that can handle the initial workload.	Incoming mail will be scanned into the EMR and routed to the appropriate doctor, nurse or staff. After the first 6–12 months, the paper chart scanning volume may drop to a level that requires fewer scanning devices.	$1,000–$10,000 per high volume scanner
Software	EMR Application	EMR application licenses allow access to a set number of users based on the actual user count or provider count. The EMR application licenses may be for full access or partial access depending on the vendor. License fees vary widely based on the target market for the EMR and staffing composition. For example, some EMRs are licensed by a provider, but only allow a certain number of users for each provider.	Licensing fee strategies vary widely by vendor. Definition of a provider license can dramatically impact the cost. Some EMRs are sold by module with discounts given for packages.	$2,500–$4,000 per user
	Scanner Software	Some EMR vendors include the scanning software in the base EMR price. Many vendors charge extra for scanning software.	Scanning software may be licensed differently from the EMR application.	$500–$1,000 per user
	PMS Interface	A separate interface may be required for the demographic information, appointment schedule and charge interfaces between the PMS and EMR systems.	The interface between the EMR and PMS may require a separate server. In addition to EMR interface costs, the practice may have to pay for PMS interface modules.	$3,000–$10,000 per interface per system.
	Equipment Interface	The practice may have diagnostic equipment that could be interfaced with the EMR. The equipment interfaces may transmit an order from the EMR to the diagnostic equipment and download the results.	May require upgrades to the diagnostic equipment and/or an interface module from the diagnostic equipment vendor.	$3,000–$5,000 per diagnostic device with an interface.

Continued from previous page

Comprehensive Working Budget	Item	Purpose	Key Issues	Estimated Costs
Third Party Licenses		EMRs may require other software from third parties. In addition to system software, the practice may need to buy word processing, and other items.	In a document management EMR, the practice may have to purchase a variety of software products to produce the files for storage in the EMR.	0–$300 per workstation and tablet.
Services	Installation	Installation services include the installation of hardware and software as well as the setup of access to your workstations.	Installation services include hardware setup, software setup and connecting the EMR system to your network. Each workstation, tablet, scanner and other device will require a certain level of setup.	10%–30% of Hardware Costs
	Customization	Customization of the EMR may be required for certain vendors while other vendors may include customization in the sales price. Do not mistake customization for setting up user preferences. Ultimately, the practice is better off if each user knows how to maintain his specific setups and preferences (e.g., medications).	The scope of changes varies widely. The more clinical content that is already in the system, the less customization will be necessary. Some vendors will train the practice but leave customization to practice resources and third parties.	Varies Widely
	Training	EMR training includes computer-based training, classes at the vendor offices, practice office training and web-based training. Some vendors have structured training programs.	Many vendors train a small group of users who then train other practice staff. Training services typically vary in price.	40%–60% of EMR Application Costs
TOTAL EMR COSTS				
Contingency Costs	Communication Upgrades	Allow for upgrades to inter-office and intra-office communications to support the EMR.	Depending on the current level of communications and the last upgrade.	Varies Widely
	Workstation Upgrades	Allows for upgrades to workstations that are questionable in light of the EMR requirements.	May be easily determined by surveying the existing workstations.	$1,000–$1,500 per workstation
	Services	Implementation and training services are typically based on time. In many cases, you may want to include a contingency fee to allow for additional training and EMR customization.	This contingency fee allows the practice to allow for additional help in this demanding project. The estimate can be refined as the vendor proposal and practice requirements get more specific.	10%–20% of estimated services
TOTAL EMR COSTS WITH CONTINGENCY COSTS				

Your Practice Management System and an EMR

An EMR does not exist in a technological or organizational vacuum. EMR usefulness will be affected by your processes, staff and your practice management system (PMS). Your PMS can help or hinder your EMR and vice versa. The key issue is where you draw the border between what you expect from your EMR as well as how you will use your EMR in conjunction with your PMS. If you are not careful, you could end up duplicating efforts, and undermining both your clinical and billing operations.

HOW EMRS WORK WITH PMSs

Most EMR systems were designed as stand alone products that work with a variety of PMS systems. As such, many EMRs have their own demographic files, procedure codes, and—in some cases—full feature appointment schedule modules: information that is also maintained in the PMS.

As the EMR industry has progressed, many PMS vendors and EMR vendors have developed relationships to offer a complete package of software to your practice. Other vendors have developed a completely integrated EMR/PMS combination where the EMR and PMS components are inseparable.

With more than 1,000 PMS options and over 400 EMR products, a wide range of relationships exist between EMR and PMS systems. The following chart shows two technology relationships (Integrated and Interfaced Products) as well as business relationships between EMR and PMS products.

TABLE 3.1

	Description	Strengths and Limitations	Examples
Integrated Products (See Diagram 3.2)	Integrated products were designed as a single product from a single vendor. The products share information from the same database.	+ Supports reports including PMS and EMR data. + Costs may be lower since only one technology base is needed. + One set of master files is shared by PMS and EMR. − EMR or PMS product may not be best of breed.	eClnincalWorks Electronic Health Systems Intergy Med-Informatics
Interfaced Products (See Diagram 3.1)	Interfaced products exchange information between the EMR and PMS. Basic exchanges are demographics, and appointments from the PMS to the EMR. Charges are passed from the EMR to the PMS. In many cases, the interfaces are based on an industry standard called HL7 (Health Level 7). However, HL7 allows for a wide range of options. Interfaces should be tested to insure that the PMS and EMR are properly exchanging information. Interfaced products may be from one or more vendors.	+ Mostly allows for multiple EMR options for a PMS. + Interface is standard product. − User look and feel may differ between PMS and EMR. − PMS and EMR products may have overlapping features that requires careful analysis during implementation. − May obscure audit trails for charges from the EMR to the PMS. − May require separate entry of master file data (Ex. CPT/ICD9 codes) in EMR and PMS. − Software upgrades could cause interface problems. − May require additional licenses and costs for products based on different technologies. − An interface server may be needed to pass information between the PMS and EMR.	MISYS Tiger and EMR NTIERPRISE and Allscripts Healthmatics
Companion Products	Companion EMR and PMS products are interfaced by a single vendor and sold as a pair.	+ One vendor responsible for the PMS and EMR. − Vendor may not be open to other EMR options. − User look and feel may differ between PMS and EMR.	Amicore MISYS Companion

— Continued

Continued from previous page

	Description	**Strengths and Limitations**	**Examples**
Joint Marketing	A PMS vendor and an EMR vendor have a preferred product relationship. Their separate products work together through an interface between the PMS and EMR.	+ The practice may get preferred pricing. + Interface is used by other clients. − User look and feel differs between PMS and EMR.	MARS and Several EMR products.
Open EMR Options	Some PMS vendors do not have a relationship with an EMR vendor. The PMS vendor offers to develop an interface with any EMR chosen by the practice.	+ Supports "Best of Breed" selection. − Interface may be costly and used by few practices. − Practice may be on its own when dealing with the PMS and EMR interface. − Upgrades to one of the products may cause interface problems.	Popular EMR Partners include Allscripts Healthmatics, and MediNotes.

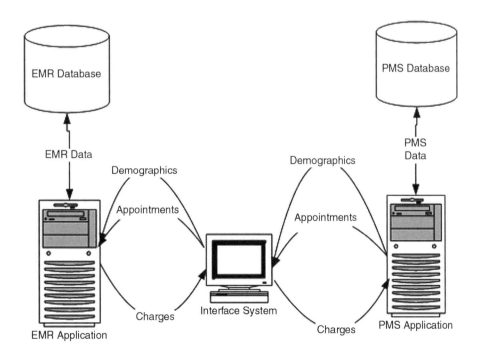

DIAGRAM 3.1—*Interfaced EMR and PMS*

Inegrated
EMR/PMS
Data

Inegrated
EMR/PMS
Application

DIAGRAM 3.2—*Integrated EMR and PMS*

All things being equal, you would rather buy a single product and deal with one vendor rather than deal with two separate products, vendors and their interfaces. However, not all products are equal. In some cases, you select an EMR that meets your need, but may not have a companion PMS offering. Some integrated products and interfaced EMR/PMS offerings have significant disparities between the sophistication and capabilities of their PMS product compared with other PMS products, and their EMR product compared to other EMR products.

EXAMPLE: You may encounter a PMS product that can handle multiple locations, but the companion EMR product does not manage audit trails and appointment activities by location. Similarly, the PMS product may not have computer assisted collection tools to manage your A/R. In other cases, the PMS may be targeted to a variety of practices, but the EMR may only have clinical content for a primary care practice.

INFORMATION EXCHANGES BETWEEN EMRs AND PMSs

Several logistical issues must be considered when you are considering an interfaced EMR. In most cases, interfaces are limited to receiving patient demographics and appointment schedules from the PMS and sending charges to the PMS. However, the practice will need a number of other data exchanges to allow PMS and EMR users to serve patients effectively and manage the practice.

The chart on pages 37 through 39 illustrates these types of information exchanges a practice would expect between an EMR system and its PMS, along with limitations to be aware of.

Some practices use EMR and PMS products that are not interfaced at all. Practices will work without an interface due to the lack of a working relationship between the two vendors/products or the costs of such interfaces. **EXAMPLE:** Some PMS vendors may not support an EMR interface with your desired EMR product. Some interfaces require substantial investments for PMS interface software, EMR interface software and a separate system to manage the interface. Be aware some PMS vendors do not accept electronic charge transactions from an EMR.

Practices that do not use interfaced or integrated products must separately enter the basic information needed by the PMS and EMR. Typically, the practice will enter the demographic information in both systems, and enter appointments for the next day into the EMR from the appointment schedule printed from the PMS. Charges are posted into the PMS from a fee slip that is used by physicians around the EMR. The fee slip is printed

TABLE 3.2

Information Type	Primary Source	Needed To	Status
Master Files	PMS	Master files include CPT codes, ICD9 codes, appointment types and other data used in the EMR and PMS systems. Some of the files are fairly standard, but other files may significantly differ between the two systems. For example, PMS products may include pricing and payer reimbursement information while the EMR merely tracks the basic CPT code and description. EMRs may maintain formulary information that must be associated with your PMS payer file. EMRs also have a number of master files that are not in a PMS including drugs, clinical database, orders, and allergies.	Some EMR vendors will load selected PMS master file data into the EMR at installation, but updates are manually entered.
Patient Demographics	PMS	Demographic information establishes the identity of patients in the EMR. Most EMR products store the PMS patient ID in the EMR demographic information. *TIP:* Although many EMRs allow you to set up demographics, you should fully evaluate how the demographic information is coordinated with the PMS. Note that not all interfaces support bi-directional demographic exchanges: the PMS may send demographic information to the EMR, but the EMR does not send demographic updates back to the PMS. A demographic link allows you to maintain consistent information between the two systems and coordinate information. Otherwise, you will be adding patient demographic information to both PMS and EMR separately.	Most EMR systems can accept demographic information from a PMS, but few PMS systems will accept demographic information from an EMR.
Appointment Information	PMS	EMRs use appointment information to track patient visits and progress. In most cases, patients are scheduled for appointments in the PMS. The appointment schedule is sent to the EMR to track the status of patients. Appointments for the day are typically displayed on the main EMR workflow screen with tasks, and to do's, patient visits and progress. Some PMSs allow patients to be checked in to flag patient appointments awaiting charges. PMSs typically do not track patient service progress (room, status) or the completion of the appointment process. PMS systems recognize a completed appointment when the charge is posted. Some EMRs track the patient throughout the visit. Medical staff determines that patients are waiting, and doctors can see which patients have been placed in a room. Internal labs, nurses, and technicians can see which patients are waiting for a service ordered by the doctor. The PMS system would only show that the patient has checked in.	Many interfaces send appointment information to the EMR, but very few PMS products accept appointment information from EMRs.

— *Continued*

Continued from previous page

Information Type	Primary Source	Needed To	Status
Payer Information	PMS	In the course of treatment, physicians and clinical staff need payer information to correctly guide patients through treatment options, locations and processes. For example, some payers may prohibit use of an internal lab or require procedures at a designated ASC. The payer information for a patient is typically included in the EMR demographic record. However, many EMRs do not necessarily maintain coverage details that may affect care options. Payer information may be used to determine prescription formularies and/or referral requirements in the EMR. Physicians may also reference insurance information to determine coverage or authorization requirements for in-office procedures. *CAUTION:* In many cases, the PMS payer codes have to be translated into a different code for the EMR. Otherwise, the EMR may not properly handle the payer specific issues and formulary.	Typically sent over to the EMR with demographic information.
Recall Information	EMR	Recall triggers are generated through clinical visits. Some EMRs allow you to generate recall notices and letters as well as track the completion of recall items through office visits. However, recall information in the EMR is not available through the PMS to assist appointment schedulers. Many PMS products have recall features to allow appointment scheduling to track recall issues. However, few interfaced EMR products send recall information to the PMS. *CAUTION:* PMS appointments will not necessarily reconcile EMR recalls or orders. Similarly, EMR plan items and orders will not be reflected in the PMS recall or appointment modules.	Typically, practice staff must separately enter the recall in the PMS. Scheduling staff may need access to the EMR to track recalls.
Clinical Orders	EMR	Clinical orders are entered by physicians/practitioners in the treatment plan for a patient. Additional orders based on disease driven protocols may be automatically generated by the EMR. Examples of orders include lab tests, procedures and other studies. Orders are needed by appointment scheduling to confirm that the patient has completed necessary testing or to schedule the patient for the appropriate type of visit in the PMS. PMS products do not typically allow for clinical order information.	Scheduling staff needs access to the EMR to track orders.

— *Continued*

Continued from previous page

Information Type	Primary Source	Needed To	Status
Surgery Scheduling	EMR	Surgery requests are communicated to the clinical support team by the doctor. The clinical support staff manages a variety of administrative, insurance authorization, testing, and facility coordination tasks to support surgery scheduling. Surgical procedures may be entered in the PMS appointment schedule, but the actual status of the various tasks associated with the appointment is normally documented in the EMR.	Scheduling staff needs access to the EMR to track surgery scheduling status. Clinical staff may need access to the PMS to manage surgery scheduling.
Charge Information	EMR	Many EMRs collect the charge information during the patient visit. Charge information is gathered when procedure and test orders are entered as well as the calculation of the E&M code at the completion of the visit. When approved by the doctor, the charges are sent to the PMS. In many interfaced PMSs, the PMS user accesses the charges from the EMR and posts the charges collected during patient service to the patient account. The PMS uses the charge information to produce patient statements and claims. In many cases, the PMS audit trail will show the charge posting person and not the clinical staff who approved the charge in the EMR. Note that many PMS products allow the user to change the posted information without creating any flag or notice that the posted charge differs from the information sent by the EMR.	The interfaces are available, but audit trails may not be clear. In most interfaces, the PMS user can edit the charge from the EMR. Some PMS vendors do not allow for charge interfaces with EMRs.
Incoming Referral Information	PMS	Incoming referral information is entered in the PMS to support claim submission. However, the doctor may need to see the referral information to determine the allowed services during the patient visit. Lacking the referral information, the EMR user will not be able to determine the specific treatment requirements. The PMS referral order will not be electronically sent to the EMR.	Doctors and clinical staff will need access to the PMS for incoming referral information.
Internal Referral Information	EMR	Doctors record internal referral information in the EMR at the time of service. Internal referrals may include a payer communication or may be directly authorized by the doctor. Internal referral information is needed in the PMS to manage appointments, file claims, and insure that you do not provide services beyond the referral.	The referral information is manually transferred to the PMS. Administrative staff may need access to the EMR system to review the original referral information.
Clinical Notes	EMR	EMRs contain the clinical record for the patient. Anyone who accesses dictation, prescription information or any other clinical information will need access to the EMR. As a practical matter this may cover a large number of your clinical and administrative staff. For example, • Payer-collection staff uses clinical notes to justify insurance claims. • Surgery schedulers need information on procedures.	Many administrative staff members will need access to the EMR.

from the PMS, and the charge information recorded on the fee slip during the patient visit. *Warning*: This workaround may lead to discrepancies between the EMR charge information and the PMS charge posting. For example, the doctor may record a certain level of service on the fee ticket before completing the clinical chart note and calculating the level of service in the EMR

> **TIP:** Do not sign the contract to purchase the PMS until you fully understand how your EMR will work with your practice management system and vice versa.

REVIEW YOUR PMS BEFORE OPTING FOR AN EMR

Take a close look at your current PMS in light of your EMR plans. Your PMS can affect the EMR options that can be practically implemented. Before beginning your search, assess your current situation. Carefully consider:

Are you Satisfied with the PMS?

Many practices are not happy with their existing PMS due to a variety of issues. The practice may have outgrown the product, or the PMS vendor may have not kept the product up to date. Unfortunately, EMRs will not necessarily improve your PMS. If your practice is not content with the PMS, then you should not attach too much significance to the current PMS in your EMR selection process. For example, you may be dissatisfied with the PMS appointment scheduler and seek a better appointment scheduler in the EMR, but a future PMS may actually be the tool used for appointment scheduling.

If you are not happy with your PMS, you should consider replacing the PMS in conjunction with the EMR implementation. Thereby, you won't compromise your final EMR selection with a PMS base that is not right for you. Additionally, you may more seriously value the integration with a PMS replacement and not limit your practice to EMR options with interfaces to your current PMS.

Does the PMS have a Preferred or Exclusive Relationship with an EMR product?

Many PMS products have preferred or joint agreements with one or more EMR vendors. Some PMS products have exclusive agreements with EMR products. If you do not choose a vendor-endorsed EMR, you may be on your own to get the PMS and EMR to interface.

> **TIP**: However, don't unnecessarily settle for the EMRs offered by your PMS vendor.

If the PMS's EMR does not include a workflow tool, or lacks features needed by your specialty, you should determine (and get the vendor commitment) when the PMS's EMR partner will address your preferences. Otherwise, you should select a more appropriate EMR product and work out the relationship needed with your PMS vendor. You do not want to compromise your EMR project to make the PMS vendor happy. You may have some leverage, since the PMS vendor would prefer to have you as a PMS customer rather than risk losing you because it forced you to go with an EMR product that is not appropriate for your practice.

Does the PMS Support EMR Interfaces?

Initially, you need to determine if the PMS product supports interfaces with EMR products. Some PMS vendors support open interfaces for any EMR vendors using an industry standard transaction structures. Other PMS vendors develop custom interfaces that are used for each EMR situation. Of course, you can always create your own interface between your PMS and the selected EMR. Some interface strategies even allow you to interface two products without the assistance of either the PMS or EMR vendor.

> **CAUTION**: Do not undertake a custom interface effort without fully understanding the implication including potential changes with future versions of the EMR or PMS, and the fact that you may be among the few (or only) practices using the combination of products.

Does the PMS Vendor Lack an EMR Strategy?

Surprisingly, a number of PMS vendors still lack an EMR strategy. These PMS vendors claim to be customer-driven and will offer to create an interface with products selected by their customers. However, some of these vendors have never interfaced their products with an EMR. Other PMS vendors have developed interfaces with a variety of EMR options, but the PMS vendor does not have extensive expertise with a particular EMR. In these cases, the costs of maintaining the interface may be spread over a few practices and be more expensive that an interface that is used by a large number of practices.

If your practice ends up developing a new PMS interface, or an interface with an EMR that the PMS vendor is not interfaced with, you will have to coordinate the work of the PMS and EMR vendors to implement the interface. The interface development effort may include designing the mechanism and strategy, as well as the specific information that will be exchanged and the sources and destinations of the interfaced data.

Interface design requires attention to a number of technical details including what triggers sending a demographic and appointment update to the EMR and the amount of time it takes to post changes to the EMR. For example, you may need the patient check-in from the PMS to update the EMR within a minute to insure that the clinical staff is adequately informed about patient flow issues.

You will not be able to benefit from the work of other practices, and you will have to coordinate changes to allow for upgrades to either the PMS, EMR or the interface. For example, a change to the PMS product appointment scheduler may change the information that is going to the EMR. You would have to test the PMS/EMR interfaces anytime you upgrade either the PMS or EMR.

Will the PMS Technology Base Support an EMR?

Most EMR products are based on a graphical user interface (GUI), such as Windows or Linux, and a database structure, such as Microsoft SQL Server, Oracle and Informix. Many older PMS products are based on old technologies and a character interface that may not easily work with your EMR selection. Similarly, you may be using "dumb" terminals that would not work with an EMR. Even if you have PCs, your PCs may not be powerful enough to support an EMR.

Upgrading your existing technology base to support an EMR could also require additional investments in the PMS infrastructure. For example, you may have to buy software to make your new PC workstations appear as dumb terminals to your existing PMS product—creating a new interface between the EMR and PMS. In some cases, you may need to pay additional money to move to a new version of the PMS, or even the next generation product of your existing PMS product.

Are Additional User Licenses Needed?

If doctors, nurses and clinical staff have access to the EMR, they may also need access to the PMS. Such access may require additional licenses fees and maybe even new PMS hardware. For example, the additional users may exceed the number of users that your current PMS hardware can manage.

The table on page 43 and 44 reveals several issues to consider when you review EMR options associated with your PMS.

Your current PMS system may pose a number of operational and implementation challenges. The key problems are based on overlapping functions and the practical implications of using an interfaced EMR.

> **EXAMPLE**: Some PMS systems allow you to scan information on insurance cards into the PMS. However, the insurance card may be needed by the clinical staff to get prior authorization or check the payer's rules. As a practical matter, a variety of information is shared between clinical and practice management processes. These issues can impact your efforts to design a workable workflow and implementation plan. In some cases, you will have to work around both the EMR and PMS vendor to determine what is best for your situation.

All things being equal, you would want to buy the EMR associated with your PMS. However, EMRs are not equal. Common barriers to buying the EMR partner to your PMS include:

PMS Upgrades—Some PMS products require upgrades to various components. For example, you may have to move to a newer version of the PMS to support the EMR interface and product. In some cases, your actually have to change to a different PMS system from your existing PMS vendor. For example, many PMS products may be sold by your PMS vendor, but only selected products (unfortunately, not your PMS) are interfaced with their EMR offering. **Hidden costs**: Upgrading your current PMS may require upgrades to your server, existing software (and new training), and, in some cases, your peripherals. You may need additional PMS modules merely to accommodate the EMR product.

TABLE 3.3

EMR Partner	Description	Issues	Recommendation
PMS integrated with EMR	The PMS shares a common database with an integrated EMR.	Integrated products frequently do not support interfaces with other EMR products.	Closely review the integrated EMR in light of your needs. If the EMR product is not appropriate for your practice, insure that you have a reliable and cost effective interface strategy. The analysis should include the cost of the interface from the PMS vendor as well as hardware needed to allow you PMS and EMR systems to exchange information.
Companion and joint marketed PMS	The PMS vendor has a standard interface with an EMR product. The EMR product is jointly sold to the practice.	The existing interface with the companion or joint marketed product may be easily used by the PMS vendor to interface with the selected EMR. The EMR vendor may support interfaces with other PMS products.	Clearly establish responsibility for the interface with the EMR and PMS vendors. Insure that the PMS vendor will not change the interface (and disrupt your interface with the other EMR product) without adequate notification. Include protections for the strategy in your contracts.
Old technology	The PMS is based on a character interface	EMRs are primarily based on a graphical user interface like Windows. If you are currently using "dumb terminals" with your PMS, these users will have to be upgraded to PCs to access the EMR.	Set up a contingency in the budget for hardware upgrades to "dumb" terminals and a technology base. Carefully review the cost benefits of the current PMS system in light of these changes. Review the design and capacity of the current technology base to identify all upgrade costs.
Unsupported or not sold	The PMS is no longer actively supported or sold. The PMS product may have been superseded by another PMS offering from the vendor or you may be using a product that was discontinued.	PMS products that are discontinued expose the practice to a sudden loss of the PMS.	Seriously consider replacing the PMS system as part of your EMR effort. Critically analyze whether to further invest in an interface that may be used for a limited time.

— Continued

Continued from previous page

EMR Partner	Description	Issues	Recommendation
Not interfaced with an EMR	The PMS is not interfaced with any EMR products. The PMS vendor says that the interface will be built for whatever EMR you choose.	The practice could easily get caught in the middle of an effort by the PMS and EMR vendors to create an interface. Your practice could end up with a one of a kind interface with the selected EMR product.	Make certain that the EMR and your current PMS provides enough added value to be worth the trouble and cost. Check into the PMS product(s) that are sold with the selected EMR. In the long term, you may want to transition to one of the selected PMS products. Indeed, you should include such an option in your contract.
Old PMS version	Your practice has skipped one or more versions and/or upgrades of the current PMS system. The upgrade(s) may have been skipped due to cost of the upgrade, costs of hardware improvements needed for the EMR and/or lack of interest by your practice.	The "upgrade" to the newest PMS version may require changes to hardware and software as well as data conversion and re-training. The costs and efforts to upgrade may not significantly differ from those of a completely new system.	Include the PMS upgrade in your technology budget for the practice. Compare the cost of PMS upgrade with implementing a new PMS.

PMS Interfaces—Hidden costs: Many PMS vendors charge for the interface module that allows you to exchange data with the EMR product. In some cases, separate charges may be required for each interface (e.g., patient demographics and appointments are considered two interfaces and charges a third interface). The interface modules may require a base charge and include a monthly maintenance fee.

EMR Features—The EMR companion product to the PMS product may not have the features you need. For example, the EMR partner for your PMS may not have the specialty clinical content you need for your practice. In other cases, the EMR may lack important features that you need, such as clinical messaging or transcription.

> *TIP*: Be especially careful to insure the EMR meets requirements that you need to effectively use the EMR. Security, audit trails and Evaluation and Management

coding tools can be easily overlooked when you are trying to fit your practice into the EMR of your current PMS vendor. In the final analysis, you should hold the companion EMR product to the same functional standard and requirements that you expect from any viable EMR product.

EMR Clinical Focus—Not all EMRs have the breadth of clinical content to address every type of practice. For example, some EMRs handle gastroenterology or ophthalmology but lack the clinical content for primary care and other specialties. And your practice may focus on a subspecialty that is not included in the clinical content of a more general specialty clinical offering. For example, a primary care focused EMR may lack the clinical content to support the cardiology specialty of one of the doctors. If the EMR of your PMS does not address your practice's clinical area then make sure you fully understand the effort needed to add the clinical content you'll need. You should be careful to itemize the scope and breadth of the clinical content needed by your practice. For example, a general ophthalmology practice will have different clinical content needs than a retina specialist. Similarly, general orthopedic clinical content may not be sufficient for a spine practice. Compare the effort needed to interface your PMS product with an EMR that addresses your clinical services "out of the box."

EMR Technology—Since many EMRs were not developed with a PMS system in mind, the EMRs are based on a completely separate technology base. Some practices find that the investment needed to buy and implement the PMS's EMR product is not cheaper (or even easier, in some cases) than buying a variety of other EMR options. For example, you may have to buy database user licenses for two databases: one for the PMS and another for the EMR. Similarly, the PMS and EMR may require a dedicated server for each module.

In the final analysis, you should not assume that the EMR partner with your PMS system is the best or less expensive strategy for your practice. Make sure that you fully understand the implications of using the PMS vendor's EMR product versus your other options.

COSTS OF CONNECTING YOUR EMR AND PMS

Connecting an EMR and PMS requires some investments in hardware and software. If the vendors have a working relationship, you must typically buy an interface module for the PMS as well as an interface module for the EMR. Such interfaces may cost from $3,000 to $12,000 or more for each interface. If you want to interface demographics, appointments and charges, you may have to buy 3 interfaces for the EMR and 3 interfaces for the PMS. Additionally, the interface may require an interface server (see Diagram 3.1 above).

Vendors that do not have a working EMR relationship will charge customization fees in addition to the purchase costs of their standard interfaces. If the vendor does not have a standard interface, you may have to invest substantial sums in a custom interface. Make sure you check the vendor's ability to accommodate other EMR products. Examine the costs to produce these interfaces, and contact customers who have such a working interface. The vendor should agree to a specific cost for any custom interfaces.

Additional interface implementation costs include technical assistance in placing the data that is being exchanged between the two systems, as well as the costs of testing the interfaces. Note that the initial loading of the data from the PMS to the EMR for the master files as well as loading the current appointments and demographic data may incur additional charges. Many interfaces will also require an annual maintenance fee.

> **TIP**: Be especially careful to insure that both the PMS and EMR vendors will appropriately support the interface and cooperate on resolving problems. Note that many of these interfaces do not post master file updates from the PMS to the EMR. You may have to separately enter the same master file record (e.g., appointment type, procedure code, diagnosis code) to the PMS and EMR systems.

Itemize the implementation costs and continuing support costs for the system that you desire. You will need to assign staff to test the interface, as well as train someone to troubleshoot the interface when inevitable problems appear in the future.

PRACTICAL ISSUES FOR REPLACING YOUR PMS

Replacing the PMS could have a significant effect on your plans for implementing an EMR. In general, most practices will want to replace the PMS before the EMR implementation effort begins. **TIP:** You need to insure that current administrative and billing operations are properly set up before you implement an EMR.

The practice needs to make sure that the replacement of the PMS is adequately accommodated in the schedule and budget for the practice. Between the effort needed to replace the PMS and settling into the new product, you may have to delay the EMR effort for 6 months to a year or more. The effect of replacing the PMS before you implement the EMR can affect the cost of the project since you may need to replace a lot of hardware and install the EMR infrastructure to move forward with the PMS.

Compiling a Practice Focused Evaluation List

The evaluation list establishes the value and significance of the EMR features needed by your practice. An evaluation list can be very extensive or very brief. Some practices use evaluation lists itemizing hundreds of criteria, while other organizations are looking to fulfill a single requirement: get a world class EMR. Although a single criterion may be too general, an overly detailed list can flood you with details and complicate your decision. Regardless of the list length, your evaluation criteria should set an appropriate standard for your EMR as well as collect information that will be used as you proceed into the implementation phase.

The evaluation list establishes the expectation of the practice for the EMR as well as the measurement standard for EMR products. Set the expectation too low, and you may end up with many products that meet the standard but risk buying a product that will not meet your needs. Set the expectation too high and your practice may end up evaluating minutia but fail to get a grasp of the product practicality. For example, some evaluation lists itemized specific data items that the EMR should accommodate without including the features needed to capitalize on the data such as a report on the pending services for a patient. In some cases, the practice may search forever for the perfect product.

Many practices spend a tremendous amount of time looking at issues that are not necessarily EMR features but are necessary. Some EMR issues that are not product specific include:

Hardware Reliability—System protection is available through the hardware server purchased, regardless of the application. Your practice can buy hardware that is vulnerable to shutdown due to the loss of a critical component or you can purchase hardware that offers redundant components. Redundant disk drives, power supplies and fans are some of the redundancies that you can purchase for your server on a cost- effective basis. For an additional investment, you can buy fully redundant server hardware regardless of the EMR software. Workstations, communications, network components, tablets, printers, and scanner selections and strategies can also control your risks without necessarily impacting your software selection.

Tablets—Tablet devices are not specific to a particular EMR product. Tablet devices can access an EMR like a workstation or work through a terminal server that improves performance for tablets in remote locations. Some EMR vendors offer a variety of tablet options that include models with and without self contained keyboards. Know that your workstation and tablet decisions are not dependent on your software selection.

Internet Access—With the right equipment and/or communications, physicians and others can access the EMR over the Internet. Some products are optimized to work over the Internet directly, while other products require a server that lets Internet users access the EMR. For EMRs that require an Internet access server, you need an internet gateway and communications services that support such a gateway (e.g., Windows Terminal Server with Citrix.) In either case, you need a practical way for the remote user to access the Internet. For example, you may install a broadband connection at the doctor's home or access the EMR from the hospital connection to the Internet. EMR access over the Internet is not dependent on your EMR software. However, the ability to access your EMR through the Internet or a remote location is not specific to an EMR product. ***TIP:*** There may be a cost difference between the two approaches, but the ability to access the EMR is not product dependent.

The important issue is to focus on the features and capabilities of the product and not the hardware and communications that you will purchase to support the EMR. Hardware and communication issues can be addressed after you have chosen the appropriate software.

EVALUATION LIST FACTORS

Creating the evaluation list is a daunting task. The first challenge is identifying the important issues and features that you need. The second challenge is articulating a concise requirement that can be used to evaluate potential solutions. To gain some familiarity with the products, you should consider looking at a few products before you compile the evaluation list.

Compiling a list of important items is complicated by your reference point, the manual patient record and current workflows. It will dramatically effect what your practice will need in an EMR. Some questions to consider in compiling your list include:

- What are the specific clinical and treatment areas that the practice is active in?
- What are the specific subspecialty area covered by the doctors in the practice?
- For primary care practices, which clinical conditions does the practice work in that would be considered outside of standard primary care area?
- What are the special aspects of the practice that need to be managed through the EMR?
- What are the supplemental services that the practice offers?
- How will the EMR be used at the front desk, clinical area, check-out and billing areas?
- What information is currently put in the paper chart?
- What supplemental information is kept outside of the patient chart?
- Where are the sources of patient information to be collected by the EMR?
- What are the testing, service and treatment orders tracked by the practice?
- What features are needed to properly serve patients?
- What information would improve the effectiveness of the PMS and administrative staff?
- Who accesses information from the paper chart and what information are they accessing?
- What are the supplemental logs, lists and diaries kept by doctors and staff to support clinical services?
- Where are copies of information from the patient chart kept? What are the copies used for?
- What is the expected patient flow with the EMR?
- What types of information and processes are involved in handing off patients among clinical staff?
- How will the EMR affect interactions with patients?

The evaluation list should highlight the issues that are important to you but not be so lengthy that you cannot practically handle or manage the list. For example, a list of hundreds of items will be difficult to evaluate and manage. Table 4.1 (see pages 50 through 69) itemizes the features that may be significant to your practice as well as the specific capabilities to look for in your evaluation. Review the table to compile an actual list in the next section.

TABLE 4.1

Feature	Significance	Look For
Basic Services		
Support	Vendors offer a varying array of support options. Some vendors offer standard working hours support with premium charges for off-hours support. Within three to six months of Go Live, your staff will probably know more about how the EMR system operates for your practice than your vendor. *TIP:* To get the most out of your vendor, consider establishing a designated support person or team that will be able to maintain "continuity of care" for your EMR. EMR vendors offer hardware support in a variety of forms. In most cases the support is coordinated with a third party support organization that the EMR vendor will contact to provide onsite support.	Support hours meet practice working hours. Emergency support on demand. One-stop handling of hardware and software issues. The practice should be able to call a single support contact to coordinate hardware and software issues. Designated support staff for your practice to maintain continuity. Specialty based support staff to address issues specific to your specialty. Annual user meetings and periodic seminars that allow you to meet other users to get ideas "from the field."
Documentation	The EMR system should be formally documented in paper and/or electronic help. Be certain that the EMR documentation is detailed enough to meet your needs. Thereby, you have a qualitative measure for any support or error issues you encounter. Note that some EMRs lack specific documentation and instructions. In some cases, the documentation consists of general information that does not contain sufficient detail to use the system. For example, the documentation may outline the screen flow but fail to explain whether the medication information is added to the patient medication list or a note is included in the E&M code calculation. **TIP:** Poor or deficient documentation may cause problems if you uncover a programming error since there may be a dispute about what the EMR does.	Clear and comprehensive documentation in electronic or paper form. Includes general directions, flow descriptions, and field-by-field explanations of EMR information. Specialty or area of medicine specific documentation that explains how the EMR works in you type of practice. Annotation notes that allows you to add practice specific instructions to the EMR documentation.
Upgrades	EMRs enhancements address evolving industry issues as well as generate new sales. New sales are needed to finance development and improvements. If new sales stop, then the vendor may start selling another product and not offer new features for your EMR system. Some vendors have specific plans and enhancement schedules, while other vendors do not release information on when the next release is or what will be in the release. **TIP:** Be wary of products that have new releases on a frequent basis. Frequent releases may indicate a new product that is still under development or has more serious structural problems. You should also be wary of vendors that have not released a new version within the past year. Lack of new versions may indicate a lack of research, development and investment in the EMR. Software releases can be costly for your practice. You may incur installation fees, disruption to operations for installation and database rebuilding, and additional training costs. The more organized the releases, the easier for you.	Review the history of software upgrades on a periodic basis (e.g., annual or semi-annually). Examine copies of release notes from recent releases. Look for enhancements and fixes. The lack of enhancements could indicate a product that is reaching the end of its marketing or support cycle. The lack of release notes may indicate a lack of planning or poor communications with EMR users. Review the release plans for the next version of the product. Note new features and look for indications that the product is making improvements and enhancements that will keep the product competitive and effective. Discuss the focus of new development by the vendor in areas of significance to your practice. Make sure that you focus on functional improvements as well as expansion of clinical content. For example, the next release may fulfill one of your evaluation list items.

— Continued

Continued from previous page

Feature	Significance	Look For
Backup Options	In addition to hardware and system backup, some EMRs are based on technologies that maintain a journal of all system activities. The backup journal may be used to update your previous backup to the point of system failure. Alternatively, the EMR technology base may support a backup hardware site. For example, the EMR vendor may send a file of the most recent updates to a remote Internet site every 30 minutes.	Maintains a backup journal of information posted to the EMR. The backup journal can be posted to update the last database backup and allow recovery to the point of the system failure. Allow for instantaneous transmission of all database activities to a backup system site. Access to a remote backup site in the event of a catastrophic loss of your system.
Security	EMR access should limit access, mobility or approval rights. Security issues are particularly important to an EMR since only an appropriate doctor or clinician can sign off on a chart note. As important, some chart notes require a physician signoff as well as a signoff from another party. *CAUTION:* Some EMR products do not differentiate between mid-level providers and doctors. If you have mid-level providers, you may need to have a separate signoff for the supervising doctor. EMR security controls will vary among practices based on size and workflow. Practices with large staffs and focused responsibilities require more specific security controls. For example, the clinical staff in the lab may be limited to lab order information and lab results entry. Smaller practices may not have a dedicated lab staff. EMR security should support compliance with HIPAA and allow you to establish access rights for groups of users. The EMR security should limit and control access to information as well as maintain the audit trails needed to monitor access issues (See Audit Trail).	A roles structure security model assigns access and entry rights by function (e.g., transcription, prescriptions, chart signing) by role or user class (doctor, nurse, technician). User roles can be defined to appropriately segment responsibility in the practice. For example, a large practice may allow a user to review a record, but not change the record. A smaller practice may not require specific controls. User roles can be supplemented at the user level. Additional capabilities can be added to a user profile and role-based permissions can be removed for a user. For example, new front desk staff may be limited to accessing only certain EMR features. Security controls access to clinical records by clinical-record area, entity, patient class and/or modality. Separate signoff authorities for mid-level providers and doctors. Supports automatic user signoff after a set-time period (e.g., 5 minutes-30 minutes). Requires user password changes within a set period of time (typically this occurs every 30-90 days). Allows users to quickly secure the screen from access, and facilitates returning to the previous EMR activity.
Practice Structure		
Entity	If your practice includes more than one legal entity, then you may be required by state and federal law to maintain separate medical records for each entity. For example, your practice and ASC may be separate legal entities that require separate medical records. Note that some states require separate medical records even for services that are provided by a single legal entity. For example, you may have to maintain a separate psychiatric file for a patient seen in a primary care practice.	Separate databases or database segmentation to keep information separate for each entity. For example, the EMR may be able to segment information by department (which could be the separate entity). An easy way for a user to switch among the entities.

— Continued

Continued from previous page

Feature	Significance	Look For
	Most EMR products are designed for a single entity. These EMR products require completely separate databases for multiple entities. Completely separate databases may prohibit sharing master file information and EMR setups as well as EMR information that is passed from one entity to another. For example, separate databases may complicate sending Evaluation and Treatment orders as well as progress reports between an orthopedic practice and the physical therapy center. **CAUTION:** Some EMR products suggest using an internal coding of the medical record to maintain separate charts. For example, ASC records start with "ASC", and clinical records start with "CLI."	Tools to transfer medical record information from one entity to another. **CAUTION:** Some EMR interfaces pass "notes" that become notes in the receiving EMR database. However, these notes do not necessarily update prescriptions or procedure lists. Mechanisms to exchange setup information, master files and customization factors among entities.
Locations, Departments and Modalities	If the practice operates multiple operating units or locations, the practice may need EMR handling by locations and departments. Many EMR products focus on the doctor and not the location or department. For example, you can see the patient appointment status by doctor but not all appointments for several doctors in a pod or department (e.g., pediatrics, internal medicine) within a location. To verify the situation in a pod or department, the manager would have to separately access each doctor's appointment list. For larger practices this strategy would not provide management tools for the office or the practice. Some EMRs track patient office location in the appointment list and may allow the user to view all patients in a pod or department. Managers can track workflow by pod or department operating units. Tracking of locations and departments may be subject to the capabilities of the PMS appointment scheduler and/or the interface between the EMR and PMS. For example, a PMS schedule with the location in a comment would not be an effective reference point for an EMR that tracks locations.	Appointment list by specific location, as well as resource. Appointment list by a selected group of doctors defined by the user. For example, all doctors using a common pool of technicians and nurses. Appointment status includes a department and/or room indicator. Room and department indicators can be easily changed. Patient status and location are easily determined. Patient status codes can be customized for the practice and location. For example, a primary care practice may want a lab status while an orthopedic practice may want to flag a patient for x-ray. **CAUTION:** Some EMRs maintain a list of rooms and status for the entire practice and not for each location. Management tools coordinate patient workflow and clinical issues by location, department, doctor and user. Management tools can display combined lists of activities for a user defined group of doctors. EMR maintains user specific routing information for patients who may be passed among several doctors and staff in the course of a visit.

— Continued

Continued from previous page

Feature	Significance	Look For
Staff Collaboration	If your practice uses a collaborative patient service model, then the EMR needs to support and track the working relationship between the doctors, nurses and other staff. For example, patient intake may be performed by a nurse who passes the patient to a doctor and the doctor turns the patient over to another nurse for treatment. The EMR should allow doctors and staff to view the patient status and situation as well as interact on the patient's situation. Some EMRs limit those interactions and will hamper your ability to capitalize on the EMR. For example, some EMRs only support a single provider that is considered the source of all EMR information. Such products will not allow you to manage additional staff or allow retrospective review of clinical information entry. All clinical information is attributed to the doctor, regardless of the source.	Routing tools to transfer patients among doctors and staff. Forwards patient records and a note from the sending party to the next responsible provider. Indicates pending patient services to the selected staff and doctors. Supports and/or requires primary and secondary signoffs of a medical record. Audit trails indicate the source of information as well as the doctor who signed the note.
Ancillary Services	Physical Therapy Centers, Optical Shops, Coumadin Clinics, Urgent Care Clinics and Ambulatory Surgical Centers are examples of ancillary services. Ideally, practices should be able to offer patients more effective services through internal services and doctors should be able to more easily access patient service information. The EMR should allow the practice to simplify patient services and referrals to the ancillary service. The internal ancillary services should be more easily accessible and better coordinated than any outside service options. For example, the ancillary services staff should be able to access the relevant patient information and the doctor should be able to review patient status.	Accepts an order for ancillary services that will be performed by internal resources. Accepts service orders. Accepts and tracks status of services for current and future visits. Tracks service order items and associated patient information. Facilitates access to clinical information needed in the ancillary area. Facilitates access to the ancillary service information by doctors and others in the clinical area. Supports messaging and patient tracking between the clinical and ancillary service areas.
Diagnostic Services	Diagnostic services include radiology, lab, and imaging departments. Some specialties, such as ophthalmology, cardiology, plastic surgery and orthopedics may have extensive diagnostic imaging capabilities. Practices with diagnostic departments will need to manage the flow of patients and orders. The EMR should support order-entry assigned to the internal department as well as the routing of patients to the department. In some cases, the diagnostic equipment can receive the patient and order information directly from the EMR. Some diagnostic equipment will send information back to the EMR or provide the EMR with a reference identifier. The reference identifier may allow the EMR user to directly access the results on the diagnostic equipment.	Accepts and tracks diagnostic service orders. Diagnostic orders can be queued and tracked by department. Results can be posted to the EMR and tracked through the review by the provider. EMR can include diagnostic images in the patient's medical record. EMR can interface with the practice's diagnostic equipment. *TIP:* You should think ahead and buy diagnostic equipment that can interface with an EMR as soon as practical. You may want to include an interface option in the purchase.

— Continued

Continued from previous page

Feature	Significance	Look For
System Setup and Support		
Personal Digital Assistant (PDA)	PDA applications are used to provide a certain level of support to physicians outside of the office. The PDA offers a limited group of functions to capture information on patient services that can be uploaded to the EMR. PDAs may support charge entry, dictation, and prescription writing. PDAs may allow for brief notes and some order information. Typically, the PDA information is downloaded into a hold area for acceptance into the EMR. Some practices implement PDA applications and never move onto a full EMR implementation. *TIP:* PDA applications may be superseded by the ability to access the practice EMR through a wireless connection over the Internet. If so, physicians could access the complete medical record on demand. This option is becoming more practical as hospital wireless networks and other wireless options become available to doctors.	Records basic clinical information, including orders, prescriptions and a clinical note. Accommodates new patient information. Accepts dictation into the PDA for posting to the EMR transcription function.
Audit Information	The HIPAA Privacy and Security standards as well as your own tracking needs require appropriate EMR audit trails. Ideally, the EMR should maintain an audit trail of entry, edit, printing, and access activities. The adequacy of the EMR audit trails may also be determined by your practice organization and patient-service style. For example, practices that use physician extenders and have many staff members contributing information into the EMR You may want to access the particular user who entered information even after the doctor has signed the note. Make sure you fully understand the audit trail that is part of the product. *CAUTION:* Some vendors have audit logs that are only accessible through system tools that are not part of the EMR application. Other EMRs only print an audit report. A number of EMR products track only the doctor who signs the chart note. Depending on your situation, you may need more accessible audit trails.	Record changes and additions are tagged with the user, date and time. Logs medical records access by patient and area/segment by user, date and time. Creates audit trails for the production and distribution of printed documents. Logs invalid security access attempts. Offers a print option to include the audit information in the patient note. Online access to audit logs with sorting and selection options for users, date, patients and information type. Includes audit log reports with user selection and sort options.
Practice Customization	EMRs offer varying levels of practice customization. Practice customization may include operational issues (e.g., Sequence of Templates), clinical content (Severity Levels), and selection options (Standard Medications). A number of EMR vendors support customization through specific programming for the practice and few "out-of-the-box" options. If your practice needs changes, the vendor will program the changes into your version of the system. Such accommodations are not the same as allowing you to select various options that are already built into the software.	Support customization of pick lists by the user. Allows for operational options selected by the practice including the order of information entry and clinical treatment standards. Allows the practice to flag clinical information that is required. Includes practice selected patient summary displays. Supports practice developed reports and documents that pull selected information from the patient EMR record.

— Continued

Continued from previous page

Feature	Significance	Look For
	CAUTION: Custom programming changes may have to be reprogrammed into future releases of the EMR. Make certain that you know how much it will cost you to keep your changes in the future. Practice-level customizations may allow you to establish EMR standards that can be further customized by users.	
Office/Location Customization	Practices with multiple offices may need to customize the EMR for the office or location. Location specific options may include patient status, rooms, task types, and procedures. **CAUTION:** Customization at the office level should be used with caution. Some office level customization could disable other EMR features. For example, office specific document types could complicate finding all radiology studies for a patient across the practice.	Supports office specific codes for patient status. Allows for office specific lists of rooms and services.
User Customization	Each user may have a different focus that should be reflected in his EMR views. For example, an intake nurse will want to see different information than a triage nurse. The surgery scheduler will need to see the list of procedures, while the billing clerk is primarily interested in dated chart notes. User customization includes information views as well as user specific pick lists for key information. For example, different providers may have specific lists of preferred medications. The user specific EMR view may be selected by the user, but many users will still need to access all EMR sections.	Maintains doctor specific codes for frequently used medications, procedures, orders by problem or diagnosis. Displays most frequently used information and templates for the user. Accepts user specific defaults for charting patient information. Facilitates quick identification of and access to templates and clinical information entry that the user most commonly uses. Allows user specific display of key patient information. Displays user specific workflow preferences (e.g., Display orders).
Interfaces		
PMS Demographic Interface	The demographic interface between the PMS and EMR eliminates the duplicate entry of patient information between the two systems. **CAUTION:** The interface may be limited to PMS and EMR structural issues. For example, a single entity EMR may not be able to offer the flexibility needed for a multi-entity PMS. **CAUTION:** An EMR may not be able to deal with a practice that uses multiple billing systems. For example, a practice may have a separate billing system for the clinic and the ASC. Multiple billing systems could result in multiple patient records and a complicated interface. Significant differences may exist between the EMR and PMS demographic information. Key information including payer codes, patient class and billing type may use different coding structures and even have different effects on the two products. For example, the patient class may drive reports in the PMS but determine drug formularies in the EMR.	Insure that combined EMR and PMS products share the same demographic information. PMS demographic information should be posted to the EMR demographic file within a minute of posting to the PMS. Verify the ability of the EMR to translate key PMS demographic codes and data into comparable EMR structures. Key demographic information includes payers, patient types, and HIPAA Status.

— Continued

Continued from previous page

Feature	Significance	Look For
PMS Appointment Interface	EMRs use appointment information from the PMS to initiate and manage patient flow in the office. Once a patient is checked in, the practice will manage patient services through the EMR. Some PMS products include a basic tracking capability for appointments. These PMSs may allow the user to check the patient in, flag that the service starts, and check the patient out. *CAUTION:* The EMR may have a competing set of functionality. For example, the PMS may present the patient co-payment requirements at check-in, but the EMR presents outstanding health maintenance items. If the PMS is used to check-in the patient, the health maintenance screening may not be dealt with until the patient is seen. The doctor may not be able to service the patient since the basic health maintenance issue (e.g., blood test, diagnostic study) was not identified at patient check-in.	PMS appointment information should be posted to the EMR within a minute of the appointment entry in the PMS. PMS check-in information is posted from the PMS to the EMR. If check-in information is not posted from the PMS to the EMR, check-in desk staff may need direct access to the EMR. EMR appointment structures and codes can be mapped to the PMS appointment features. For example, the PMS appointment type and doctor codes may have to be translated into the relevant EMR codes to properly display the appointment in the EMR. *TIP:* Use of many appointment codes to accommodate individual doctors may affect the EMR. Ideally, you should standardize the appointment types in the PMS to simplify the patient flow tools in the EMR.
PMS Charge Interface	EMRs generate charges during the clinical process. EMRs may capture charge information as procedures are performed, as well as calculate the E&M code at the completion of the patient service. The transfer of charge information should be triggered by the approval of charges in the EMR. Once the charges are approved, the charges are sent through the interface from the EMR to the PMS. *TIP:* The formulation of charge information in the EMR does not leave a paper audit trail of the charges for the practice. The lack of a charge slip for EMR services has significant operational and audit implications for the practice. The specific audit procedures will depend on the EMR-to-PMS interface. For example, some PMS systems accept the EMR charges into a hold area that can be edited by the front desk before posting. Such strategies may require additional audit procedures.	Provides an E&M code calculator to accept information from the physician and calculate the level of service. Automatically calculates the E&M code based on the EMR charting process. Maintains an audit trail of the E&M code calculation. Accumulates procedure and testing information as the patient is served in the practice. Uses standard CPT and ICD9 codes to send the charges to the PMS. Includes modifier codes with the charge transactions. The charges are passed and posted to the PMS system in time to check the patient out of the office. Includes a daily charge report that can be used to verify PMS posting.
Lab Interface	To improve efficiency, and avoid problems, the EMR should have an electronic interface with your key reference labs and/or lab information system. Some EMRs will interface directly with the lab equipment. Lab orders are entered in the EMR during the patient visit. Orders can be electronically transmitted to the appropriate lab system. Thereby, the doctor can view outstanding lab orders and status through the EMR.	Verify that the EMR can submit orders electronically to key reference labs (e.g., Labcorp, Quest Diagnostics) or in-house lab system (e.g., LabDaq or Orchard LIS.) Verify that the EMR can receive results electronically from your key reference labs and/or lab systems (e.g., LabDaq). Electronic results should be maintained in a hold status until the results have been reviewed.

— Continued

Continued from previous page

Feature	Significance	Look For
	Results are accepted from the reference or internal lab into the EMR. Results are saved to the patient chart for review. The EMR should track the review status of incoming lab results (e.g., pending, performed, received, reviewed, signed).	
Diagnostic Equipment Interfaces	As the repository for all chart information, the EMR should accommodate information and/or images from diagnostic equipment. Diagnostic equipment interfaces accept information directly from the equipment into the EMR. If the diagnostic equipment can generate an electronic record, then the information could be loaded into the EMR though an interface or saved as a standard image (e.g., pdf, bmp). Standard images can be saved as an EMR image. If the diagnostic equipment does not produce an electronic record, then the printout can be scanned into the EMR. The practice should insure new diagnostic equipment can be interfaced with the EMR. **TIP:** Any diagnostic equipment purchased by the practice should include an interface with the EMR. Additional interfaces with the EMR may require additional interface purchases from your EMR vendor. Some EMR vendors charge a set fee for each interface even for interfaces with equipment that has not been previously interfaced with their EMR. Other vendors charge a substantial amount of money for any new interfaces. Such interfaces could represent a substantial investment for the practice. **NOTE:** A number of EMR systems will store pointers to diagnostic images on your diagnostic equipment. The pointer is used to open the file using the diagnostic equipment's own software.	Compile a list of the current diagnostic equipment at the practice. Offers a variety of interface options including direct interfaces, and including a standard image file in the EMR record. Determine the availability of an interface between the practice's diagnostic equipment and the EMR. Develop an interface strategy for each type of diagnostic equipment.
Partner Interfaces	Some practices have electronic interfaces with a variety of business partners. Electronic interfaces could include downloads of information from a hospital, or other provider. For example, you may be able to download radiology reports from an imaging center. You may need to download results for a hospital lab.	Interface toolkit that simplifies and manages electronic exchanges of information including images. Offers a practical service to interface with other parties. Accepts downloaded clinical information for review and posting to the patient's EMR chart. Supports interoperability exchanges of data using standard transactions such as the continuity of care record.
HIPAA		
HIPAA Privacy Standards	HIPAA Privacy Standards address the handling and management of protected health information (PHI.) Practices are required to maintain information on the authority to use and disclose PHI. The EMR is the practice's repository for PHI.	Maintains information on patient consent forms and status. Allows for limitations to be documented. Accepts a signed patient HIPAA consent or disclosure form that can be viewed through the EMR.

— *Continued*

Continued from previous page

Feature	Significance	Look For
	To guide practice staff, the EMR should control and track access to EMR information (See Security and Audit Trails). In addition to the consent form, the EMR should allow for highlighting and tracking any limitations as well as information on authorizations and disclosures. Disclosure tracking may include a log that the user fills out or an EMR audit trail. *CAUTION:* Some PMS products include basic information on consent forms. However, few of those products manage other aspects of HIPAA Privacy.	Supports information on authorizations for disclosure of PHI. Accepts information on disclosures of patient medical information. The information may be manually entered by the user or electronically generated by the EMR. Maintains an audit log of printed and faxed information from the EMR. See Security and Audit Trails.
HIPAA Transactions	HIPAA Transactions include several standards that apply to an EMR: Continuity of Care record includes key patient identification and problem information for patients that are being referred to another practice. Additional Claim Information Transaction supports the exchange of clinical information, such as supporting documentation for claims or encounter reports to collaborating practices. Service Review Transaction includes information on referral authorizations, pre-certifications and pre-authorizations. Retail Drug Prescriptions could support exchanges with pharmacies. Although few clinical HIPAA transactions are being exchanged today, support for HIPAA Transactions and other EDI will become an increasing important EMR issue. At a minimum, the practice should understand the vendor's plan to support the EMR-related transactions.	Produces and accepts Continuity of Care records containing key patient information. Generates Electronic Prescriptions from the EMR to a clearinghouse and participating retail pharmacies. *TIP:* Make sure that the electronic prescription service is connected to the key pharmacies in your area. Generates outgoing HIPAA Transaction Service Review referrals to payers. Posts incoming HIPAA Service Review referrals, pre-certifications and pre-authorizations to the EMR. Produces outgoing HIPAA Transaction Additional Claim Information for selected EMR information.
HIPAA Security Standards	HIPAA Security Standards allow for administrative, physical and technical safeguards for protected health information. Several HIPAA Security issues are addressed in the Security and Audit Trail Features.	Locks medical record to prevent any changes. Simplifies access and research of audit logs for access and updates to the EMR. Vendor offers a disaster recovery service.
	Patient Information	
Patient Information Entry	Patient information entry accepts patient information directly into the EMR. The patient may enter the information through a Web Site, directly into a workstation (that has been secured from other EMR functions) or scanned in on a "bubble form." For Internet Entry, the patient is provided with a special code to enter information for posting to the EMR.	Accepts initial HPI information through the Internet. Accepts Social and Family History through the Internet. Accepts Refill Requests through the Internet.

— Continued

Continued from previous page

Feature	Significance	Look For
	TIP: Patient interactions through a Web Site is gaining wider acceptance among patients. *CAUTION:* Some EMRs have a Web Portal for Messages, but the information is not accepted into the patient's electronic chart. *CAUTION:* Split vendor systems may pose problems for taking full advantage of patient interactions. For example, the patient would have to go to one portal to pay your bill and a second to submit a question for the doctor. Typically the doctor or nurse can review the information before the patient data is posted into the EMR. The doctor or nurse can correct and enhance the information as needed.	Supports Message Exchanges between Doctors and Patients. Identifies the information entered by the patient. Accepts information from the patient or another party (e.g., parent, guardian). Includes an indicator for the source. Information can be vetted and reviewed before posting to the EMR. After posting to the EMR, the actual source of the information can be viewed from the EMR.
Access Patients	The EMR will manage all patient interactions and services are well as act as a repository for your clinical information. A variety of options should be available to facilitate access to the patient by demographic information as well as access to the patients with a scheduled appointment or outstanding issues. Direct access to patient information from the list of appointments and/or tasks ensures the user is accessing the right patient information. EMRs that rely on an external email facility to manage patient issues and flow may not offer a direct connection to the electronic chart.	Accesses patients by name, medical record number, SSN, office and primary physician. Provides a list of patients based on appointment dates. Appointment lists can be viewed for date, location, provider and/or status. Presents list of patients with outstanding issues and to-do's. The EMR should facilitate access directly to the patient chart and/or document those who do. Tracks the status of current to do's and maintains a repository of previous practice efforts and to do's.
Patient-side Notes	The practice may need to highlight an issue that is not otherwise noted in the medical chart. The issue may be a continuing problem or a temporary issue associated with the patient visit (e.g., patient service issue). The EMR should allow for a patient alert to be maintained between patient visits, as well as a temporary issue that is only relevant for the current visit. For example, a patient who is discharged from the practice may get a special patient alert to indicate the discharge.	Establishes patient alerts that are displayed when a patient is accessed in the EMR. The alert can be customized for each patient. Supports a miscellaneous note on a non-clinical patient issue that is not saved in the patient chart.
Recalls	PMS systems support a basic recall capability. PMS systems may allow you to define a recall note and/or recall type that is entered with a recall date. Some PMS products also present the recall when an appointment is made. However, PMSs do not track whether the recall was actually fulfilled through a specific clinical action. EMRs may accept the patient return purpose and timeframe when entering the patient plan. However, this information is not commonly available in the PMS. In addition to the recall information, some EMR products maintain clinical treatment standards that are de facto recalls. The clinical standards in many respects are more powerful and useful than a recall.	Displays patients with recall instructions in the clinical plan according to user-selected parameters. Tracks completion of clinical recalls with appropriate clinical events. Generates general recalls for patients meeting a select clinical criteria based on diagnosis and specific findings. For example, a recall could be generated for all cataract patients without a visual field test in the past 12 months. Supports clinical standards that will be automatically assigned to a patient based on age, sex and conditions defined by the practice. For example, a cardiologist could establish an automatic EKG warning for all at-risk patients as well as patients older than a certain age.

— Continued

Continued from previous page

Feature	Significance	Look For
	For example, a clinical standard for a blood test in an EMR will only be fulfilled by the completion of a blood test. Non-EMR based recall systems do not typically track the completion of the recommended test or treatment.	
Clinical Chart Setup		
Clinical Content	Clinical content includes the specialty or primary care specific clinical information that is accommodated by the EMR. The clinical content that comes with the EMR may include a set knowledgebase of clinical findings, specific disease state templates and other clinical setups. Some products have a very specific clinical focus, while others offer a wide range of clinical content. For example, some EMR products focus on cardiology practices while several products are only sold to orthopedic practices. Note that the types of existing users will be a good indicator of the EMR clinical content. In the event that the EMR does not have clinical content for your treatment area, the vendor may offer to develop the clinical content or present the advantages of setting up your own clinical content. **Beware:** The setup effort may represent a substantial level of commitment. If you can find the clinical content you need, then you significantly mitigate the risk of failure.	Collect existing clinical forms. The practice should verify that the most common conditions are accounted for in the EMR clinical content. Itemize the various clinical areas and modalities that the practice will need covered in the EMR. *TIP:* Make sure that you include the specialties and sub-specialties that the practice works with to clearly define the clinical content. Review the EMR clinical content relevant to the practice. Ensure that the supporting clinical content includes documenting the clinical issues, access to additional clinical details and generating a relevant clinical report. **CAUTION:** You should not assume that your sub-specialty is covered if the vendor claims to cover the specialty area. For example, a product that has otolaryngology clinical content may not necessarily have audiology content.
Documentation Standards	EMRs can support the use of disease-based documentation standards. Documentation standards may be enforced through requiring entry of selected data and/or retrospective analysis of completed patient records. Documentation standards may also be managed with EMRs that calculate the E&M code from the data entered. If adequate information is not entered, then the code level will be affected. For example, the lack of a chief complaint could clearly be highlighted when the EMR calculates the E&M code.	Requires entry of selected information at the practice's option for selected conditions and templates. Reports on signed patient charts that do not meet the documentation standards.
Clinical Toolkit	Many EMR products include software tools to develop customized screens, lists, documents, or templates. The EMR toolkit allows the user to select the specific data items and entry options on the template. For example, the items to record a breathing problem could be selected by the user. EMR products that do not include a clinical toolkit may offer customized programming services.	Using a screen or template builder, the EMR clinical content can be customized by trained practice staff. Adding clinical findings to the knowledgebase by end users on demand. Document generator supports patient specific information into a letter produced by the EMR.

— Continued

Continued from previous page

Feature	Significance	Look For
	CAUTION: The vendor may reserve the right to make changes to improve the product and/or marketability of the EMR. Thereby, a serious practice issue may not be resolved if the resolution would not be applicable to a wider array of practices. Some EMR products are sold as is without customization tools. Even if you are pleased with the product now, it may be difficult to change the clinical content as you gain experience with the EMR and your practice changes.	Vendor demonstration on building a basic template or screen of information that you use in the practice. **CAUTION:** Insure that the template builder requires a level of technological competency that the practice can support. For example, some tools require little programming skill, while other toolkits are designed for use by a dedicated programmer.
Addendum and Amendments	Many practices are concerned with the permanence of a signed and un-editable EMR record. As a practical matter, the practice may need to revisit or amend the EMR record to account for test results or new information provided by the patient after the EMR note has been signed. The EMR should allow authorized users to amend the signed EMR note. The amendment may take the form of an additional note at the end or beginning of the note or changes that are actually entered within the clinical note. The previous information and changes should be clearly identified.	Addenda can be added to chart notes or existing notes can be annotated. Images can be annotated with a drawing tool. Changes to previous notes can be clearly identified. Maintains the content of the original note. Maintains information on original and subsequent contributors to the clinical note.
Patient Summary Screen	The patient summary screen presents the key information needed for a patient. Summary information options include procedure lists, user preferences, outstanding tasks, image lists, encounter lists and chart note lists. Some EMR products have a static patient summary screen, and others allow the practice and/or user to select the summary contents. Patient summary options are useful since different practices may focus on different information. For example, a pediatrician may want to see immunizations while a surgeon immediately want to see the list of previous procedures. User specific summary options accommodate the clinical focus of various staff members and doctors. For example, the intake nurse may be interested in vitals and medications, while the surgical scheduling staff may focus on outstanding orders and the last visit note.	Verify summary screen includes key information on the current patient situation. Review the options for patient summary screen displays. Test the ability to navigate from the summary screen item to the relevant clinical item. Determine the sort and filter options for the patient summary information. Sort options may include date, item description and modality. Filter options may include selected dates and doctors. Verify the patient summary screen can be customized for users. The customization options should facilitate access to relevant information based on your practice staff. For example, a technician may need to see only the orders, vitals and current medications.
Clinical Charting		
Charting Patients	To minimize transcription and improve E&M coding, the EMR should be used to chart clinical records at the time of service. The look and feel of the EMR should be reviewed to ensure that the doctor and staff can easily navigate through the clinical content to chart the appropriate note. Ideally, a sample note from the practice should be used to test the charting process.	Practical screens to enter clinical data at the time of service. Support for WNL (within normal limits). Starting chart notes based on previous visits. Entry of structured chart notes using templates. Accepts as ad hoc notes and documentation.

— Continued

Continued from previous page

Feature	Significance	Look For
		Variety of documentation tools including templates, notes, drawing tools and reference materials.
		Allows for dictation into selected chart note sections.
Treatment Plans	Treatment plans are sequences of clinical services that are designed to address a specific condition. For example, a series of office visits and diagnostic tests over a 3-month period may be used for a patient with pneumonia. Treatment plans are patient specific. Most doctors will want to start off with a template for frequently encountered issues for the practice and modify the treatment plan for the patient's specific situation.	Accepts patient treatment data including procedure, performing provider and required date/delay period. Accepts a standard treatment plan that can be assigned to and customized for a patient. Treatment plans can be tracked by patient. Treatment plan items are separately managed for completion.
Clinical Protocols	Some EMRs manage treatment standards based on clinical protocols. The protocol can trigger treatment messages based on a variety of factors, including sex, diagnosis, risk factor, procedure and age. For example, a female patient older than 40 should have periodic pap smears and mammograms. The clinical protocols should be defined by the practice according to specialty and treatment standards. The clinical protocols should be verified with all patients who meet the protocol criteria, to catch issues that may not be triggered by treatment plans and recalls. Some EMR's will test the protocols on a periodic basis (Ex. Weekly) while other EMR products test the patient against the protocols on demand or when you access the patient's electronic chart.	Maintains practice specific treatment requirements based in diagnosis, age, sex, previous procedures and patient history. Tracks performance of treatment requirements by patient. Highlights clinical protocol issues for patients automatically. Reports on overdue clinical treatment protocols.
Transcription	A transcription facility with the EMR is important to most practices. In some cases, the scope of the EMR project is to make transcription available through the EMR. Other practices continue to offer a transcription option to doctors after other physicians are charting with the EMR. As a practical matter, you may continue to offer transcription for items that cannot be built in to the clinical content, such as extensive chief complaints and detailed analyses. The transcription facility should support tracking of the transcription process from dictation through distribution to outside parties. Some EMRs allow the user to insert voice dictation fragments into the EMR. The voice fragments are routed to transcription and inserted into the EMR chart note.	Accommodates a completely transcribed note or a brief insert into the clinical note. Accepts and tracks a voice (.wav or wave) file with the dictated note. Tracks status of transcription from entry to edit, approval and distribution. Identifies transcription without review by the doctor. Supports distribution of the transcripted document. Maintains a list of distributed documents. Accommodates working with a remote transcription service.
Image Storage	Every practice needs to store and track images, otherwise, a shadow paper file will be needed for non-electronic information (e.g., diagnostic images, ER reports, diagnostic reports).	Image classifications facilitate saving and locating images based on an image type and encounter date. Image description can be entered by the user.

— Continued

Continued from previous page

Feature	Significance	Look For
	EMR images may be stored with limited or extensive information. Some products merely assign an image type to the image. Other products allow for a free text description. A few products accept user specific indices that can vary by image type. For example, you could enter the hospital for a radiology image and the payer for a letter.	Practice specific indices (e.g., hospital, payer, study date) can be associated with the image description. Stamps each image with user, date and time. Images are listed in the several sort orders including by image type, date of service with other documents and user/doctor. Image status identifies images that are pending review by a doctor or other party.
Image Management Tools	EMRs will store images as they are received by the practice. Practices that scan the patient paper chart will store the original paper chart as an image group. The paper chart storage is a difficult challenge since paper charts were never designed to be scanned. The image management and annotation tools of the EMR will allow you to get the most out of your paper record images. Other images stored in the EMR include images from diagnostic equipment and incoming paper documents that are included in the patient's chart.	Image batch sorting tools allow reorganization of images. Image thumbnail viewer. Supports multiple image types including BMP, PDF, DICOM and digital camera images. Rotates images. Supports annotation of images with drawing tools. Pulls images out of one image file to save with updated annotations. Supports drawing on an image and saving the image with the annotations. Images can be printed within the associated clinical note
Insurance Benefits Management	An EMR allows for entry and assignment of diagnostic and lab orders by the physician. However, some payers limit the studies that can be performed in a physician office. **CAUTION:** EMRs that include insurance coverage management are subject to the interface with the PMS.	Tracks insurance coverage limitations by payer. Notifies doctor on order entry of insurance coverage limitations. Supports ABN signature.
Medication Entry	On patient intake, current patient medications are recorded. Current medication information may be incomplete or lack specifics. For example, the patient may not know the strength of the drug. EMRs should accept the information for other prescriptions at whatever level of detail is possible. **TIP:** The EMR should also accept the doctor and clearly differentiate between practice prescriptions and prescriptions from other practices. **CAUTION:** Some EMRs mix the patient medications list with the practice prescriptions. The mixing may impact the production of summary reports on prescriptions written.	Records information on medications from other providers with and without details. Accepts information on the prescribing physician. Medications are considered for drug interaction when new prescriptions are entered. Clearly differentiates between reported medications and prescriptions issued by the practice.

— Continued

Continued from previous page

Feature	Significance	Look For
Prescription	EMRs enable the production and documentation of prescriptions through a single process. Information entered as a prescription automatically is included in the clinical documentation. The same information is used to print, electronically transmit or fax a prescription. Typically, a preferred list of drugs can be maintained with the SIG, dosage and strength. The doctor can prescribe a drug from the doctor's preferred drug list, a list of drugs based on the patient's problem, or access the complete list of drugs from a third party drug database, such as MediSpan. In some cases, EMR vendors maintain their own drug database. Prescription information is stored in a separate table for each patient. Previous prescriptions can be accessed to record and manage refill requests from patients. Some systems support updating the original prescriptions. Other EMRs will generate a new prescription with a reference to the original script. In some cases, EMRs create an entirely new prescription without a reference to the original prescription. Reports can be produced to track prescribing patterns. Prescriptions written in the EMR may be subject to formularies by payer.	Accepts prescription information that is maintained in a list of patient prescriptions. Presents drugs based on disease state, provider favorites and/or frequently used drugs. Offers standard prescription orders for a doctor. Supports recording distribution of drug samples. Works with a drug database (e.g., MediSpan, First Data) that includes drug information. Highlights payer specific drug formularies. Considers allergy and disease interactions. Drug utilization review considers drug interactions. Submits prescriptions by fax. Supports electronic scripts (Ex. Surescripts.) Accepts and monitors refill requests. Discontinues prescriptions with a reason.
Lab	Lab orders entered in the EMR are used to document the patient plan as well as create a trackable order. Lab order information typically includes the lab test, current or future date and performing lab. Lab orders are tracked by the EMR through order, specimen capture, results receipt and results review. Incomplete, and/or overdue lab tests can be identified for follow-up. Operationally, the practice may need to check incoming lab results to ensure that all of the information is available for a patient visit.	Accepts lab orders including the date expected. Prints labels for specimens. Allows for tracking of labs performed by the practice as well as external reference labs. Tracks status of various lab steps: order, entry, draw, results and results reviewed. Highlights abnormal results. Supports electronic interfaces with reference labs or an in-house lab information system. Displays time series results in table and graph form.
Procedure Orders	Procedure orders include the in-office procedures that may be performed by the physician or other staff. The entry of the procedure is used to document the treatment plan as well as trigger service performance. The procedure may be performed by the doctor or other staff members. The procedure results will be documented in the EMR and included in the patient record. For future procedures, the EMR should facilitate tracking if the procedure is completed. The EMR should support locating incomplete procedures.	Accepts procedure orders for a current or future visit. Manages status for in-house and outside procedure orders including order entered, pending, scheduled, performed, and denied. Supports patient consent forms and signature directly into the EMR associated with the procedure order. Delegates the procedure to other staff and tracks procedure status and progress.

— Continued

Continued from previous page

Feature	Significance	Look For
	TIP: Many EMR products assume that the procedures will be performed during the current visit. Make sure that the product can handle future activities without distorting the current visit note.	Supports authorizations and consents for procedure orders. Includes documentation tools for procedures. Identifies outstanding procedures.
Diagnostic Studies	Diagnostic studies are currently recorded in the paper chart and supported with a written prescription. EMRs accept diagnostic studies as part of the plan for the visit. The entered study can be used to route the patient to the appropriate practice department or print a prescription. **TIP**: Many EMRs assume that the study will be performed in your practice. If you refer patients to outside parties for studies, the EMR should differentiate between studies performed internally and externally. The EMR should track the status of the diagnostic study and support completion of the study upon review of the diagnostic results. The diagnostic results may consist of a message, incoming note or scanned image of a report. The EMR should track outstanding reports and practice staff should be able to easily identify diagnostic results needed for the next patient visit.	Accepts current or future diagnostic study orders. Tracks recurring diagnostic study orders. Prints prescriptions for diagnostic studies performed by other healthcare organizations. Manages status for in-house and outside diagnostic studies, including order entry, scheduled, performed, report received, report reviewed and report approved. Orders are tracked until fulfilled by the receipt, review and acceptance of the results. Supports authorizations for procedure orders.
Patient Education	Currently, preprinted patient education items are distributed to patients as needed. In some cases, the patient education items are bulk-printed documents from various organizations and, in other cases, the patient education is printed by the practice. EMR-based patient education materials can use a wide array and range of materials. In addition to computer-based content from a subscription service, you may be able to add practice developed materials and items from other sources. The EMR may support producing the education materials directly from the EMR and recording the distribution activity as part of the clinical record.	Includes a database of clinical patient education covering the practice's area of medicine. **TIP:** Make sure that you check the breadth and depth of the clinical content in light of practice services. Allows for practice developed patient education. Supports customization of patient education content for a specific patient situation or clinical condition. Documents distribution of patient education materials to a patient. Supports online patient education products and demonstrations.
Surgery Scheduling	The surgery order and scheduling process involves coordinating clinical and administrative tasks for a patient. Surgery scheduling tasks include pre-surgery testing, medical release, consent forms, payer authorization, physician scheduling and facility coordination. Currently, practices use a form to track the surgery schedule status. Unfortunately, numerous clinical and administrative staff must compete for possession of the patient surgery scheduling information or keep their own copies of the surgery form. The surgery scheduling information is an important component of the EMR record.	Accepts a procedure order with diagnosis for a future surgery. Includes a note area for doctor preferences and surgery details (Ex. Anesthesia, type of implants, etc.) Tracks user defined action items and issues to complete the surgery scheduling process. The action items can be customized for each patient, and include insurance, facility and clinical issues to support surgery scheduling.

— Continued

Continued from previous page

Feature	Significance	Look For
	The list of surgery items and status should be maintained in the EMR. Then all of the staff involved with patient scheduling can track the status of each patient surgery through the EMR.	Surgery action items can vary by surgical procedure. Scheduling features support surgery scheduling, including appointment location, appointment note, appointment status (to flag completed surgery scheduling versus pending surgery scheduling efforts) and wait-list appointments. Supports patient consent forms and signature directly into the EMR associated with the surgical procedure.
Product Sales and Distribution	A number of practices may sell products to patients to support treatment and clinical services. For example, dermatologists may sell skin treatments, pediatric practices may sell lactation supplies and orthopedic practices may sell DME. The EMR should record the product as part of the treatment plan and manage the associated charge posting to the PMS.	Maintains a list of products sold by the practice. Records product sales in the EMR as part of the treatment plan. Passes relevant transactions for posting to the PMS. Includes reports to support inventory tracking and usage. Tracks inventory usage and levels.
Quality Reporting	PQRI and other quality reporting requirements are generated from clinical data. PQRI standards from Medicare include deterministic items as well as items that may require research. By capturing the quality reporting factors through the EMR, practices will be able to easily review the backup for the reporting items.	Supports entry of PQRI quality measures in the EMR. Sends the quality reporting codes to the billing system with the charges.
EMR Workflow		
Patient Flow Management	Patient flow management includes tracking the patient status and location. Typically, the user can maintain several pieces of data in the patient appointment list such as location, status and/or a comment. In some EMRs, the user sends the patient chart to the next user with a note or instruction. Some EMR products do not adequately support the flow of patients in the office. In some cases, vendors suggest the use of a dummy paper chart for each patient in the office or a flag/light system for the office. Unfortunately, this strategy does not allow the practice to optimize operations or develop the management strategies available with computerized patient flow. For example, a paper "token" to manage patient flow will not keep management informed of any bottlenecks or delayed patients. An EMR workflow tool allows managers to view patient flow from another location or for all offices in the practice.	Includes a list of scheduled appointments and patient status (e.g., arrived, roomed, in service, checked-out.) Doctors and staff can pass a patient to another party with a forwarding note. Doctors can monitor status of their patients in the office. Records current status and location of a patient to facilitate patient services by doctors and staff. Maintains an audit trail of patient flow activities for management review. Presents management level views to monitor current practice patient flow.

— Continued

Continued from previous page

Feature	Significance	Look For
	Patient flow tools should include a location, department and practice-level views to allow managers to monitor patient flow and proactively address problems	
Workflow Tools	An EMR informs the doctors and other clinicians on the wide range of patient issues and visit activities. The EMR must manage and support tasks and messages including patient messages, patient office movements and staff services. In a collaborative patient service environment, physicians and staff need to be able to check on the status of a particular patient as well as the status of a doctor's schedule. For example, patients queued for radiology services are important to the radiology department, the doctor who sent them and the PA awaiting the results and returning patient. Office managers may review real-time office status to manage patient flow and allocate resources.	Task management accepts information on patient specific and general items for users. Maintains information on patient status that can be viewed at the patient, department (e.g., lab, radiology, diagnostic testing) and doctor levels. Includes a manager function to monitor task status and performance. Displays overdue tasks. Supports performance tracking including tasks completion statistics, tasks by status category and time to complete tasks.
Task Management	A paperless office must manage the same avalanche of incoming issues and paperwork found in the paper-based physician office. Telephone messages, incoming results and documents and miscellaneous patient related queries must be recorded and tracked. An EMR is superior to paper-based messaging since the task is attached to the patient EMR chart upon entry. Some EMRs also maintain a direct connection to the appropriate document. For example, an incoming radiology study will be directly accessible. The message or task instantaneously appears on the user's workstation. When the user has a few moments between patients, the clinician or doctor can select the task; instantaneously access the patient EMR chart or incoming item. Tasks can dramatically cut the response time to patient inquiries and issues.	Supports task information including message, task type and priority. Assign tasks to a particular user or a group of users. Forwards tasks to other users or replies to the originator of the task. Allows for tasks to be completed at a future date. Monitors task priority and due date to inform appropriate parties and management.
Sign-Off	In many situations, other staff may enter information or serve patients that require physician signoff. For example, a PA may perform a post-op exam that is signed off by the physician.	Assign staff authority to enter notes but not sign the notes. Supports signing authority for different levels including doctors, and mid-level providers.
	The sign-off capability enables the use of triage strategies and mid-level clinicians. The appropriate staff treats the patient and the medical record is automatically forwarded to the doctor. The EMR enhances patient service and supports the use of physician extenders. **CAUTION:** Some EMR products do not differentiate between the signing of a chart by a doctor or a mid-level provider. **TIP:** Some EMRs combine the signing authority with the audit trail. In these cases, the signer is assumed to be the source for the entire note.	Presents unsigned notes for sign-off by designated doctor or supervisor. Displays unsigned note list for doctors and practice management.

— Continued

Continued from previous page

Feature	Significance	Look For
EMR Analysis Tools		
EMR Reporting	Discrete EMR data is a specific finding or data item that is accessible to a reporting program. For example, a temperature data item with a value of 100 can be reported if you select all temperatures higher than 99 degrees. However, a note that says "patient temperature is 100" may not necessarily be found with certainty. *TIP:* Searching for discrete information within text is not as accurate as seeking specific data items. A reporting feature should allow for generating detail or summary reports for patients meeting a user-defined selection and sort criteria.	Supports graphing of flow sheet information. Custom reporting of patients based on selected clinical data including patient summary data and chart details. Presents active patient list screens to access relevant patient records. Offers flow sheet option for selected clinical data. Generates lists of selected patients in user defined sort and grouping orders. Produces statistical reports based on user selection criteria and reporting formats. For example, total prescriptions by drug for a selected date range.
Quality of Care Factors	The EMR should provide tools to track, manage, and analyze the clinical information. Forms and knowledgebase EMRs may maintain specific information on patient conditions and services. To capitalize on the information, the EMR should provide tools to analyze and check the clinical records.	Requires documentation standards for clinical conditions. For example, the EMR allows the users to require entry of vitals for primary care visits. Supports clinical documentation surveys to determine clinical records that may not meet compliance and/or treatment standards. For example, a list of patients on Coumadin without a blood test during the office visit could be produced. Supports statistical surveys of patients who meet a specific clinical condition and services panel.
Collections support	The practice must supply clinical records in support of claims on a frequent basis. Payers may require documentation for certain E&M codes as well as procedures and other selected services. In the absence of a paper chart, the insurance collections staff will need access to the clinical record. The EMR should support quicker access to the clinical information needed to support claims.	Supports read-only access to selected EMR information. Easily creates clinical note with patient identifying information for claim justification. Allows information to be directly faxed from the EMR to the payer with a cover note. Maintains a log of faxed information and destinations.

— Continued

Continued from previous page

Feature	Significance	Look For
Clinical Reporting	In the absence of a paper chart, all outgoing reports are produced from the EMR. The EMR collects a large amount of discrete information on a patient visit, but outgoing documents may include only a limited or selected amount of clinical information.	Clinical reports can be generated with selected information or all information according to a user option. Clinical reports include information from the clinical note as well as prescription, order and other EMR information. Allows information to be directly faxed from the EMR to the selected party with a cover note. Maintains a log of faxed information and destinations.
Letter Writer	Using discrete data, the EMR can generate letters with selected information. For example, the practice could design a letter with information plug-ins that report on a particular aspect of patient care or that it's time to make another visit. *TIP:* Some EMRs pull the entire clinical note into a word processor for editing. The user would edit the letter, and then save the letter in the EMR as a separate document. However, letter editing can lead to inconsistent presentation and incorrect information (e.g., deleting a critical word.)	Includes a self contained letter generator based on clinical information. Maintains an audit trail of distributed letters and the letter contents.

PRACTICE AREA SPECIFIC EVALUATION CRITERIA

In addition to general requirements for an EMR and the specific clinical content needed by your practice, you should also consider features that are specific to your specially or practice area. Table 4.2 (see page 70) presents some of these features.

CREATING THE EVALUATION LIST

The evaluation list should consider the factors and issues described in the preceding sections. You should create a specific list that includes the nuances of your practice as well as general EMR requirements. For example, you need to insure that the EMR includes clinical content for your specific clinical services and area. A primary care practice with cardiology and OB/GYN specialists will not be satisfied with general internal medicine clinical content.

The Evaluation List is used to record the feature analysis of the EMR product. The analysis may consist of the following columns:

Feature—Features itemize the specific requirements for the practice.

> *TIP*: Strive to be as specific and concise as possible. The features should be structured to evaluate all of the selected products. Be careful about

TABLE 4.2

Practice Area	Features to Look For
Allergy	Accommodates allergy testing. Supports serum formulation and tracking. Quickly documents allergy shots. Tracks shot treatment programs.
Cardiology	Tracks device use by patient. Supports stress tests. Manages Nuclear Camera Studies. Accommodates Cath Lab. Includes Coumadin Clinic Management.
Dermatology	Manages and Tracks Biopsy Results. Supports Product Sales. Documents in-office procedures. Accommodates Anesticians.
Gastroenterology	Stores colonoscopy results. Manages long term recall for screening colonoscopies.
Endocrinology	Supports specialized growth charts.
Internal Medicine	Includes sufficient clinical content for doctors in selected specialty areas. Supports sick patient visits. Tracks compliance with well patient services. Manages outgoing referrals.
Neurology	Interfaces with EEG testing equipment.
OB/GYN	Tracks prenatal care trends. Tracks pregnancy progress. Supports mammography results. Manages tracking patients with abnormal pap smears.
Oncology	Manages Chemotherapy Regimens. Tracks Inventory and Treatment Preparation. Supports Administration of Treatment.
Ophthalmology	Interacts with Optical Product Sales. Coordinates with Optical Lab Work. Supports Contact Lens Sales and Fulfillment. Accommodates ASC Services. Interfaces with Diagnostic Equipment.
Orthopaedics	Interfaces with a PACS system. Tracks Evaluation and Treat Orders. Accommodates ASC Services. Supports Physical Therapy Services. Supports Occupational Therapy. Tracks DME.
Otolaryngology	Manages working with Audiologists. Supports Audiograms. Supports Hearing Aide Sales. Manages Hearing Aide Service.
Pediatrics	Handles Sick and Well Child Conditions. Easy handles ad hoc "family" add ons for a patient visit. Maintains Immunization Information. Supports Lactation Counseling. Tracks Immunization Standards. Includes Growth Charts.
Radiology	Interfaces with a PACS system.

using terminology or features that will tilt the evaluation toward a specific product. Consider the following feature composition suggestions:

Simplify the Requirement—You should balance the need to keep the number of evaluation features manageable with your need to practically score the item. A focused feature will have a limited number of measurable aspects. For example, a feature that states "supports medications from other providers, sample drug distribution and refills" will be difficult to review and score. The feature could be split into 3 different items and include more details about each of the three aspects.

Avoid the Trivial—Many requirement lists include items that every product needs to have, and are basic requirements. Trivial items create a lot of work, may obscure the product differences and inflate scores. For example, a patient name, and address may not be as significant as the ability to annotate a clinical image.

Eliminate Common Standards—Although few products do everything, you should minimize the commonly available features that are included in virtually every product. For example, the existence of diagnosis, procedure, provider and patient files are common standards for EMRs. These items are needed to support other features.

Articulate the Practice Need—The features should clearly identify the practice needs and not include items that are not relevant. For example, one practice has the doctors performing all patient services without physician extenders. A simpler workflow feature should be used. If a practice has a very specific workflow requirement, it should include the specific workflow item in its feature's list.

Include Required Components—The feature may include the specific manner in which you want to handle a specific item. For example, a practice with some new diagnostic equipment may include specific interfaces with the specific vendor equipment in the feature list.

Minimize Specific Design—The features should avoid specific design issues and strategies, unless the design is a feature requirement. For example, you may require customized templates without dictating the tools to support the templates.

Evaluation—The evaluation assigns a feature score for the reviewed product. The scoring scale can be based on any system you are comfortable with. You could use words (e.g., None, Poor, Fair, Good, Excellent), characters (A, B, C, D, E), or numbers (1–10). However, you should be careful to use a scale that can be easily used and summarized. Steer away from a finely graduated scale. For example, a score with 15 different gradients may have such fine differences, that the scoring and interpretation will be difficult to determine. Summarization is best done with a numeric scale. Indeed, practices that use non-numeric scales frequently convert the scales to numeric values to arrive at a total score. An easy scale to measure the capability of a product follows:

0—Does Not Support the Feature—The EMR does not have the feature you desire. If the vendor currently lacks the feature but is releasing the feature in the next release, you should still award a '0,' but note the coming enhancement in a comment.

1—Does Not Fully Support the Feature—The EMR partially provides the feature but is missing a significant component. In many cases, the partial fulfillment is based on a workaround in the EMR. However, you should be certain that the workaround is practical and actually useful.

2—Fully Supports the Feature—The EMR fulfils the feature in a straightforward manner. If there are any questions on the feature, review the handling and capabilities again.

3—Exceeds the Feature in a Meaningful Way—The EMR product contains an additional capability that enhances the EMR in light of the practice's needs. The evaluation should not include an enhancement that is not significant to the practice. The additional capability should be documented in a comment.

Importance—Importance prioritizes the features in your evaluation. Although each feature may be significant, some features will be more important than others. For example, the interface with a specific PMS product may not be important to the practice, if you are not happy with the current PMS. Importance can be assigned any scale you wish subject to the scoring issues for the evaluation. A scale to consider follows:

4—Critical Requirement—The lack of the feature would prevent the practice from meeting its EMR goals. For example, the lack of a workflow feature would undermine the usefulness of an EMR in a collaborative practice. Practices that have a unique workflow style may require features that support the current workflow.

3—Important Requirement—The feature is needed to achieve operational efficiency. For example, the inability to track incoming patient appointments may require PMS system appointment management by clinical employees.

2—Nice to Have—The feature would help the practice but is not a key requirement. For example, some specialty practices may not need clinical recall features.

1—Optional Requirement—The feature is not necessary for the practice to use the system. For example, the interface with the PMS for charge entry may not be as significant for practices that have complex coding and modifier posting issues.

Comments—After spending a significant effort evaluating products, most people find it difficult to recall the specific capabilities of the product. To preserve key information from you review, consider recording a brief note for each feature. The note should indicate the key reason for the evaluation score. For example, you may include a note with a "0" evaluation that the vendor promised the feature would be in a future released. A comment for a "1" evaluation may state that outside providers are not entered in the medications' list. A "2" evaluation comment may state the workaround used to meet the requirement. A "3" score may be accompanied with a note that the EMR product is the companion product to the current PMS.

The following table presents a template for your own Evaluation List. Below it is an example of an evaluation list. *Caution*: This example should serve only as a starting point for you to develop your own evaluation list, not as your complete list. There will be specifics about your practice that should be taken into consideration in modifying this list.

TABLE 4.3

Feature	Evaluation	Importance	Comment

TABLE 4.4

EMR REQUIREMENTS	Evaluation	Importance	COMMENT
General Technology and Business Issues			
1. Support - Vendor should offer a full range of support services including hardware, software, and training.			
2. Ease of Use - Product should be easy to use and easily accommodate the needs of individual users.			
3. Audit Controls - Maintains adequate audit trails and allows access to the audit trails.			
4. Security - Access is controlled at the system and user level.			
a. Security can be based on user-defined groups of users.			
b. Access can be restricted at the functional level (i.e., prescriptions).			
5. Privacy Standards - Existing Features Support HIPAA Privacy Requirements.			
6. Security Standards - Existing Features Support HIPAA Security Requirements.			
EMR Patient Access			
7. Interfaces with Practice Management System (PMS) - The EMR accepts demographic and patient scheduling information from the PMS.			
8. Access Options - Patients can be accessed by Account Number, Patient Name, and Chart Number.			
9. Schedule Access - Patients can be accessed through a list of patients who have checked into the office. The access list tracks the patient from check-in to check-out.			
Clinical Records			
10. Images - Stores images and scanned correspondence for reference.			
11. Practice Specific Records – Practice specific screens with clinical information can be established and maintained.			
12. Content - Clinical forms, images, and content supports clinical practice areas.			
13. Patient Summary Screen - Key patient information is displayed in a user definable screen to highlight clinical issues and needs.			
14. Patient Questionnaires - Accepts information from patient questionnaires into the medical record.			

— Continued

Continued from previous page

EMR REQUIREMENTS	Evaluation	Importance	COMMENT
15. Transcription Tracking - Tracks transcription from entry to approval and distribution.			
16. Prescriptions - Accepts patient prescriptions and monitors refill activities.			
a. Accommodates prescriptions from the practice and other doctors used by the patient.			
b. Records drug samples.			
c. Tracks refills.			
d. Includes online information for drugs and dosages.			
e. Supports online formularies by insurance company.			
f. Maintains preferred drugs based on physician and/or diagnosis.			
g. Tracks interactions.			
h. Supports electronic, faxed, and printed prescriptions.			
17. Lab			
a. Exchanges Orders and Results with Reference Labs.			
b. Manages the status of lab orders.			
c. Accepts and tracks results from the lab. Supports alarms and/or flags for critical values.			
d. Supports flow sheet views of lab tests.			
18. Procedure Orders			
a. Tracks Procedure Orders.			
b. Prints Procedure Order for Outside Provider.			
c. Prints patient information on preparing for the procedure.			
d. Manages the status of a procedure order.			
19. Diagnostic Study Requisitions			
a. Tracks requisitions for diagnostic studies by practice departments and other providers.			
b. Prints Order for Outside Provider.			
c. Manages the status of diagnostic requisitions.			

— Continued

Continued from previous page

EMR REQUIREMENTS	Evaluation	Importance	COMMENT
d. Stores diagnostic images.			
e. Electronically interfaces with diagnostic equipment.			
20. Patient Education			
a. Prints patient information from a handout library or customized items.			
b. Maintains a log of distributed information in the patient's medical record.			
Workflow Support			
21. Office Flow - Records the progress of a patient or issue (i.e., refill request, lab results).			
a. Supports dated "to do" lists with future ticklers.			
b. Patients can be transferred between doctors, clinical staff and clinical units.			
c. Supports Physician Sign-off of Medical Records from services provided by mid-level staff.			
d. Addenda and notes can be added to patient records.			
22. Facilitate User Activities - Includes features that help users identify pending tasks and patient service items.			
a. User desktop helps manage patient service items (Ex. Messages, Reports)			
b. User desktop manages patients in the office.			
23. Charge Transfer - Charges can be transferred from the EMR to PMS.			
Management Reports			
24. Graphs - Graphing tool allows trend and comparison graphing of clinical information.			
25. Clinical Based Patient Searches - Supports searching for patients matching treatment and/or diagnosis.			
26. Report Writer - Users can define custom reports by selected content, records, and sort criteria. Information queries can be based on demographic and clinical information.			
Letter Writer			
27. User Letters - Clinical information can be merged into a user-defined letter.			
28. Log and Image – Sending logs and images of letters sent are maintained by the system.			

Selecting Products to Review

With more than 400 EMR products and a steady stream of new EMR offerings, the options present a daunting task for the average practice. In some cities, you may have dozens of EMR vendors competing for your business. Some practices spend years looking at systems and options without making a decision. Many practices look at a wide range of products and cannot differentiate between the products reviewed. In many cases, you find an exhausted staff with little to show for their effort.

Before selecting products to review, you need to consider several initial filtering strategies to cut the number of EMRs and focus your effort. Much like any other product, a particular EMR product will not satisfy every practice. Some EMR products are focused on a specific specialty or on primary care. Other EMR products are designed for practices where the doctor independently serves the patient. A number of EMR products are appropriate for a practice based on size alone.

IDENTIFYING CANDIDATES

Once you have decided to explore an EMR, you will be quickly inundated with materials and sales people for a variety of EMR products. In larger cities, you will encounter dozens of options. Indeed, you will be contacted by a host of new vendors as you proceed through the selection process. Your current PMS vendor as well as perspective PMS vendors will be soliciting your business. The current PMS vendor will seek to capitalize on their existing relationship with your practice, and prospective PMS vendors will be seeking to get on the short list to serve all of your technology needs.

Identifying potential candidates should be a fairly open process to insure you will consider products that are of interest to your staff and doctors. In essence, you are trying to identify viable products as well as preemptively address questions that will surely arise as you proceed in your decision making process. When you come across a vendor, you should catalog the vendor name and briefly evaluate the appropriateness of the product for the practice. In many cases, you will be able to quickly eliminate the product. However, you should document the rational for the decision to not seriously consider the product.

You will not necessarily take a detailed view of all the products, but include the products in your list of EMRs that your could look at. In general, you will come up with 8 to 15 different products that people in your practice, local, or specialty area are talking about. You can gather potential solutions from the following sources:

Systems of Interest to the Doctors and Key Staff—Practice staff and doctors are an excellent source of information on potential EMRs. EMRs are a hot topic among practices and healthcare industry professionals. Doctors and staff members may have seen one or two products that piqued their interest. You should account for the products that are being discussed by your physicians and employees. If you account for these systems, and fairly consider potential options, you may be able to avoid "buyer's remorse" after you make your decision. Presenting thoughtful reasons for not reviewing a product will instill confidence in the process and gain credibility for your final decision.

Colleagues in Your Area—Local practices are good sources of information on EMR vendors. Local practices can help you identify EMR products sold in your area, as well as the support capabilities of the vendors. You will probably encounter a local EMR vendor with a limited install base that is used by a local contact. **TIP:** Make sure the local vendor has a viable product before you consider the EMR for you practice. For example, the product should be used in a practice that is of similar size and/or services. Many such initiatives are still in the development stage and may require your advice to develop and your expertise to test the capabilities of the EMR.

Colleagues in Your Specialty—Other practices in you specialty area can help identify products that as sold to organizations in your specialty. Be especially careful to verify the specific subspecialties and services that the other practice provides as well as their ancillary offerings.

Colleagues in Practices of Similar Size—Similar size practices can help you identify the types of products that are used in practices of your complexity and volume. For example, a practice with more than one legal entity will need a more sophisticated EMR selection and setup. Similarly, a multi-office practice has a number of coordination and management issues that are not issues for practices with a single location.

Systems Supported by Hospitals—A number of hospitals are offering EMR products to their medical practices who work at the hospital.

CAUTION: These initiatives vary widely from buyer discounts to an entire EMR system controlled and managed by the hospital. In some cases, you control your EMR and in others, the hospital makes decisions for your practice. In any case, you want to check into these options. In the event that you buy into am EMR solution that is controlled and managed by the hospital, make sure that you have a clearly defined exit strategy in the event that the hospital leaves the EMR business at a future date, or your practice changes. Looking back on the problems some practices encountered when some hospitals shut down their MSO organizations, an EMR exit strategy is prudent and necessary to protect your practice and your patients.

TIP: Practices that have relationships with more than one hospital should carefully evaluate the implications of following one particular strategy. Indeed, some practices are being torn between the conflicting and differing product offerings. Do not try to use more than one EMR product for your practice. Such an approach may make your hospitals happy, but undermine your practice operations and services.

TIP: In any event, you should make sure that you end up with an effective solution for your situation regardless of the preferences of the hospital(s.)

Systems Supported by Key Partners—Some local associations or regional healthcare networks may uses or endorse an EMR vendor. Be careful to fully consider the product situation in your analysis. For example, some groups may back a particular EMR to encourage adoption among their members to improve their physician networks. In other situations, you may find out that a referral fee is being paid for your business.

CAUTION: Some physician networks are requiring use of a particular product as a condition of participation. Note the conflicting problems discussed about hospitals apply to other practice relationships.

But before you go too far with whatever a key partner may be using, quiz the partner on these two elements:

Selection Process—You may discuss the EMR selection process and how they chose the product. The other products considered and their final decision will help you refine your process and focus. For example, they may have eliminated a product for an issue that does not apply to you such as the influence of a closely related healthcare organization. In other cases, they may have bought a system for a reason that is irrelevant to your practice.

EMR Status—In some cases, practices may be in the middle of installing a system or have yet to fully deploy a product. For example, one closely related practice of an internal medicine practice was "completely installed and operational" when in fact only a single doctor was using the EMR to chart his patient visits. The EMR report was printed out and placed in the patient chart. The current status of the implementation can tell you what may be a good candidate as well as which strategies will not work in your implementation.

At the end of collecting potential products, you may have eight or more EMR products that you could consider. Next, focus on the products that have a good chance to meet your needs.

SITUATIONS TO AVOID

With the large number of existing vendors, the number of new and evolving entries is surprising. New products are coming out from a variety of companies. Although you may be tempted to buy into a new product or extension of an existing product for a number of reasons, make sure that you are fully informed of the level of effort involved and what, if anything, you will get out of the investment. *Here are 5 warning signs to be wary of.*

1. Small Installed Base–

Dozens of products have small numbers of installed systems. The vendor may have few installations due to the nature of its target market, continuing development, and/or early product lifecycle issues. In some cases, the EMR business is ancillary to the main business of the vendor. For example, some PMS vendors have sold a limited number of companion EMR products. The PMS product is the main business, and the EMR merely rounds out the product line.

These vendors have been successful implementing and supporting a limited number of EMR installations. In some cases, the small installed base allows the vendor to focus attention and resources that have been significant attractions to the EMR customers.

In these situations, you need to concern yourself with the longevity of the vendor and how long the business can operate with limited revenues and resources.

> *TIP*: In the event that you resolve to purchase a system with a limited number of users, make sure that the contract protects your practice in the event that the product is not viable in the long run.

2. Develop an EMR product–

A number of physicians and practices feel that there are no adequate EMR products. The PMS and EMR market clearly proves this point. The initial development of many of the more than 1,000 PMS, and 400 EMR products was initiated by a doctor who was frustrated with the products available in the marketplace.

If your practice cannot find the right product, you may be tempted to get involved with the development of a new offering. Typically, the practice teams up with a software developer to design a new product. In many cases, the software developer is new to healthcare.

However, the development of an EMR product can consume a significant amount of resources and time. EMR product development cycles of 2 or more years are not uncommon. During that time, you will be expected to provide subject matter expertise, testing resources and even real life testing support for the new product.

Unfortunately, at the end of the process, you may not end up with a marketable product. Even if you successfully complete an EMR for the practice, you are not assured that other practices will buy the product. The final product may specifically reflect the needs and operations of your practice, but may not be sufficiently flexible to work for other practices. In the end, you risk having a customized system that is only supported and maintained by and for your practice.

> *TIP*: Before undertaking such an effort, verify that the new EMR product will represent a dramatic competitive advantage for the practice. Thereby, the risks associated with creating and maintaining a custom product will be offset by overwhelming benefits to the practice and patients.

3. Enhance the EMR Product–

Some practices get involved with an existing EMR product that requires substantial enhancements and changes. The changes may include adding features practices want, or repairing mistakes from the initial implementation. For example, an EMR product may lack a lab module for practices with internal labs. *Beware*: Some EMR products lack drawing tools and imaging modules. A number of EMR products do not include workflow or patient health management tools.

Enhancing an EMR product can be even more complex than creating a new product. Initially, you need to catalog the necessary enhancements to meet the needs of your practice. The software publisher needs to analyze the changes and determine a workable way to add the capability to the EMR. The practice and EMR vendor have to agree on the specific implementation of the enhancements, timeframe, and, in some cases, cost. Unfortunately, changes may add complexity and appear awkward. For example, you may have to access another screen to enter additional information that is not part of the current EMR.

Regardless of the out-of-pocket costs, the EMR vendor will frequently look to your practice to define the changes and collaborate on the design, development, and testing effort. Depending on the level of enhancements, the effort could consume a lot of your and your staff's time. Do not underestimate the time that you may need to support the design of the enhancement and the extensive amount of time needed to test the changes. For example, adding additional information to the patient intake screen would require testing of the data within the screen as well as the effect of the date on the exam documents, E&M coding and even the follow-up list of patient services.

4. Develop Clinical Content–

Some EMR products may have a reasonable functional offering, but have not been implemented in your specialty. Typically, the EMR is in use in a primary care practice, but has not been installed for your specialty. The clinical content for your specialty may be present at a very high level, but the depth of details needed by a specialist is not available. In other cases, a product targeted to a specialist may lack the breadth of clinical content needed to work in a primary care environment.

The practice will be expected to work with the EMR vendor to improve the clinical content to support the specialty, sub-specialty and/or primary care clinical areas. You will be expected to develop clinical content that comprehensively addresses the specialty/primary care area in a manner that could be applied to a wide range of similar practices. If you are a sub-specialist, you may need to develop content that you may not typically use. For example, a hand surgeon may have to develop general orthopedic content before adding the hand surgeon subspecialty.

The EMR vendor will rely on the practice to provide subject matter expertise, develop the content and support the testing of the clinical content. In some cases, the practices may be expected to support marketing to other practices for compensation based on sales. These issues may be part of the contractual obligation of the practice and often complicate the negotiations of a contract. For example, your practice may be obligated to support marketing activities and allow your name to be used in advertising.

Before you agree to support the enhancement of clinical content, make certain that the basic functionality and capability of the EMR meets your needs and that the resulting clinical content will be worth your investment.

5. Market Segmentation–

The practice marketplace is highly segmented, and, in some cases, highly specialized. Practice structure, size, patient service styles and other factors determine the capabilities of the EMR. As such, you should be very wary of EMR products that do not have a presence in your type or size practice. The product may lack features, clinical content for your clinical area, and even operate in a way that will not work in your practice. For example, interfaces with diagnostic equipment may be an important factor for your practice, but the EMR's target market may not have such equipment.

The lack of comparable practice installations may lead to offers to enhance the product or enticements for your expertise to customize the EMR. However, these offers should be critically evaluated in light of the level of effort that you will have to invest in the development effort and the scope of the development effort.

> **CAUTION:** Before committing to any product that will require your expertise and time, you need to clearly understand and define the level of effort that the practice and the vendor will invest, as well as what the end product will look like. In the final analysis, the decision to use a product with these issues may be a great benefit to your practice. However, there are many practices that have pursued similar initiatives without achieving the goals and results they expected.

In the final analysis, the less you have to do to make the product work for you, the better off you are. For example, you may be better off going with a product that meets your needs than buying into the development of a product that requires additional work. However, in the absence of an appropriate product, you should not avoid situations and products that will provide you with a substantial benefit and competitive advantage.

PARING DOWN YOUR EMR PRODUCT LIST

Completing a detailed analysis and review of every product that you identify will be an expensive and time-consuming task. Even if you were to review all of the products, your selection team would have difficulty remembering the specific capabilities of each product reviewed. To pare down the list to viable candidates, perform an initial analysis of the potential products.

As you analyze the product options to pare down the list, you should keep notes on why each product was not further considered and the rational for not performing a detailed review. Then you can account for options and be prepared to itemize why a particular product was not granted a detailed look. The documentation will come in handy when your doctors and/or staff review the selection process, and/or query on the viability of a particular product. Consider the following 4 issues to reduce the list to potential vendors:

1. **Practice size**—A number of selection criteria depend on the size of the practice. Location management, workflow tracking, and patient service issues can be significantly impacted by the size of the practice. When you initially consider a product, determine if the vendor has installed his product in existing practices that match your size and structure. The key criteria would include the number of physicians, staff and locations. Taking an EMR in use in a solo practitioner's office and trying to use that same product in a 7-doctor practice with a couple of physician extenders runs a number of significant risks. Key questions:

   - Is the EMR used by practices with a similar number of providers and staff?
   - Does the EMR have current installations with as many or more locations?

- Do the EMR practices use similar ancillary and diagnostic service offerings?
- Do other EMR users have the same type of staff and doctor composition?
- Do other practices use the same type of clinical support strategies for the doctors?

2. **Clinical Areas**—Some EMR products focus on selected specialties and/or types of primary care. Clinical focus may determine the types of features as well as the specific clinical areas covered by the EMR. For example, a primary care focused EMR may lack surgery scheduling support. You may even uncover a number of odd nuances depending on the original practice that started the clinical content. For example, an ENT focused product may lack audiology documentation tools and not accommodate hearing aid orders. Key questions:

- Which specialties does the EMR currently serve?
- What are the specific subspecialty areas covered by the EMR?
- What are the specific services or disease states that current EMR practices focus on? For example, a sports medicine practice would have different needs than a general orthopedic practice.
- What ancillary services are supported by the EMR?
- What diagnostic services are supported by the EMR?
- What products are distributed by the other practices?

3. **Patient Service Style**—EMR systems are built around one of several different patient service strategies. Some EMRs are structured as the personal documentation tool of the doctor. The EMR assumes that the doctor records and approves all information. Some EMRs assume that the patient is initially seen by a nurse, and then treated by the doctor. Not all EMRs support patients being handed off between ancillary services, diagnostic services and other staff during a patient visit. If the practice uses physician extenders and has a wide range of patient services offered in various practice departments, you need to verify that the EMR will support your patient follow strategy before you invest a lot of time in a detailed analysis. For example, one practice purchased an EMR that did an adequate job of documenting a visit, but assumed that the doctor would call the nurse in to transfer responsibility for a patient. The practice was using an EMR top document with the old flag system to manage patient flow. Key questions:

- What is the model patient flow strategy supported by the EMR?
- Do the EMR audit trails include tracking of a collaborative patient service process?
- Does the EMR support the various types of clinical staff and doctors involved in patient service?
- Does the EMR facilitate supervision of mid-level providers working under a designated doctor?

- What is the assumed EMR process for incoming patient issues, such as messages, follow-up, and test results?

4. **PMS Interface**—Depending on your PMS situation, you may want to insure that the EMR product includes an established interface strategy for your PMS. You can choose to require an existing interface with you PMS product or a mutually workable strategy. For example, some PMS and EMR systems have interface toolkits that support standardized interfaces with other products. **CAUTION**: Some EMRs and PMSs only interface with selected partner products while other EMR vendors have established a toolkit to interface with any PMS product. **TIP**: If an EMR product does not offer an interface strategy, you should seek out other EMR options. Key questions:

   - Does the EMR have a standard interface with your PMS?
   - Does the EMR receive demographic information and appointment data from PMS products?
   - Does the EMR send charges to PMS products for posting charges?
   - Does the EMR support additional data exchanges with the PMS?

Notice that price is not listed as a major qualifier in the selection of EMR candidates. Price driven decisions do not insure that you will get value for your investment. In too many cases, practices primarily qualify EMR solutions based on the "cost of the system." However, without completing an analysis of the product and its pricing structure, you will not be able to determine the real cost. For example, a cheaper or basic EMR without the tools to manage your workflow, or allow for images of documents, may be substantially more expensive with the necessary modules. **TIP**: The mix of purchase and support costs can also distort a cost-based criteria. For example, a product with a low acquisition cost but higher annual support cost may be more expensive than a product with a higher acquisition cost, but a low annual support cost.

At this early stage of your search, vendor estimates are based on general assumptions and unspecific estimates. Many vendors will present a general quote based on some undetermined estimate. Such quotes lack any realistic basis for you practice and make untenable assumptions. For example, a practice with various mid-level staff could be facing substantial additional charges for vendors that classify mid-level staff as fully licensed providers. The analysis of initial cost estimates are hampered by a number of factors including . . .

- A less expensive EMR that does not allow you to support a paperless operation may require continuing paper medical record costs.
- Significant issues are not included in a preliminary estimate. Without a detailed proposal, you will not be able to determine a realistic delivered cost for any product. Important components that could be easily missing from any preliminary quote include conversion services, appropriate licensing, diagnostic equipment interfaces and additional software.
- Vendors significantly vary in their pricing strategies and options. A focus on license costs could be ancillary to significant differences in support, training, and service

costs. For example, an inexpensive license fee could be offset by more expensive support fees from the vendor. Such fees could offset any license cost benefits in the first few years of EMR use.

- Half of the costs for a typical EMR in the first 5 years are attributed to hardware and support fees. In many cases, buyers focus on the license fees and installation fees and exclude significant cost components. For example, some vendors include the first year of support in the license fee while other vendors start charging support fees when the system is delivered.
- Time based services are frequently used for support and implementation services. Usage based costs reflect the standard implementation services that the vendor provides without considering your specific situation. **TIP:** A vendor that includes fewer hours is not necessarily a cheaper system. For example, the vendor is not in a position to include integrating their system into your current computer network until the current equipment has been analyzed in light of the EMR hardware requirements.
- Service and hardware exclusions distort the true cost of many vendors. Vendors may have varying degrees of costs for key services and hardware issues you may need for your EMR. **Beware:** For example, off-hours implementation and training may be charged at premium rates for practices that want to work on EMR implementation outside standard working hours. Similarly, an EMR Vendor with extended service hours may prove cheaper than a vendor with additional charges outside of a shorter standard service hour window.

In general, pricing concessions in the negotiation for purchasing an EMR can frequently cut the cost differences between competing products. For example, vendors may offer discounts for larger number of users, significant hours, or products bought at the same time. Indeed, comparable products are frequently priced within a fairly narrow margin. **TIP:** Product cost differences will only become clear when you take the time to specify your needs to insure the vendor includes all of the hardware, software and services needed for your EMR effort.

After you have focused your attention on a couple of viable EMR products, you can proceed to get workable proposals and evaluate them to produce a comparable cost comparison.

4 EMR PRODUCT TYPES

Not all EMRs are created equal. EMRs are based on a couple of underlying strategies that can have a substantial impact on your implementation and use. EMR products come in several different models:

Document Management

Document Management EMRs are designed to work with other products that develop the clinical information. The finished information is tracked and managed by the Document Management EMR. For example, you may use Word to document a patient visit, or a drawing tool to document a patient condition.

As you are saving the document or image, you invoke the Document Management EMR which allows you to associate the document/image with a patient record, description, and/or date. In some cases, you can assign specific information to a document. For example, you may be able to assign the hospital to a procedure report. Examples of document management EMRs include *SRS*, NG Cabinet and TouchChart. **TIP**: Some EMR vendors will sell the document management module as a standalone product.

Document management systems may actually store the file with the clinical information within the document management database, or save a pointer to the file that you have created. The original file may be accessed through the document management system, and, in some cases, the original software used to create the file (e.g., Word).

In some cases, document management based EMR strategies are used with paper-based forms to collect new patient information. The patient form is scanned into the document management systems to add information to the medical record. Of course, document management EMRs could also accept documents from other applications and documentation tools. For example, you could use a drawing tool with an image of your existing intake document to fill out an electronic version of your intake form. The intake form could be saved in the document management product.

EMRs that support paperless medical records include a document management feature. A sample screen from the document management module of Sage Intergy EMR follows (see Figure 5.1).

FIGURE 5.1

Forms

Forms-based EMRs use a screen-design tool to create a checklist like a typical flowsheet or intake form used by many practices. Instead of checking boxes on a paper form, the Forms based EMR allows you to define the screen based on your existing forms or some other standard. Some forms-based EMRs allow conditional handling and data entry. For example, data entry may differ for male and female patients or the form could automatically trigger the printing of a prescription when you check a drug in the treatment area. Similarly, a Forms Based EMR could automatically date and time stamp the template and print a consent form for a patient procedure.

Forms-based EMRs may be particularly attractive to practices with an extensive base of flowsheets and precise clinical workflow requirements. Depending on the capability of the form design tools, you can program specific activities, and workflows directly into the template. For example, an intake record could automatically generate the lab task for a patient that meets certain clinical data entries. The template could be programmed to conditionally trigger the lab test, and route the patient.

Some forms-based EMRs are programmed by the vendor only, and other products include tools that can be used by practice staff. Some knowledgebase EMRs include a form-building tool to support a specific checklist for the practice.

Most forms-based EMR vendors offer specific clinical content for selected specialties and clinical areas. Additional clinical content may be available from third party and other practices. NextGen EMR and Centricity EMR are examples of forms-based EMRs. A sample screen from NextGen, a forms-based EMR is shown in Figure 5.2.

Knowledgebase

Knowledgebase systems use extensive lists of findings or conditions to document patient visits. The most widely used knowledgebase is Medcin. Medcin contains over 300,000 items that the user can choose from. Several other knowledgebases exist, and some vendors design and maintain their own knowledgebase. Of course, selecting findings from such a list is a massive undertaking.

To simplify the use of the knowledgebase, knowledgebase EMRs include a variety of tools and classifications to focus your selection. For example, most knowledgebase EMRs include search tools that help you locate findings based on keywords as well as organizational structures to categorize findings into clinical areas. Knowledgebase EMRs include user-defined lists, and, in some cases, templates of findings that allow you to organize the findings you most commonly use.

Knowledgebase EMRs generate documents from the findings into SOAP structures, and/or user-defined letters.

A4 Healthmatics, Electronic Healthcare Systems, Purkinje, and Allscripts Touchworks EMR are examples of knowledgebase EMRs. A sample screen from Healthmatics EMR is shown in Figure 5.3.

FIGURE 5.2

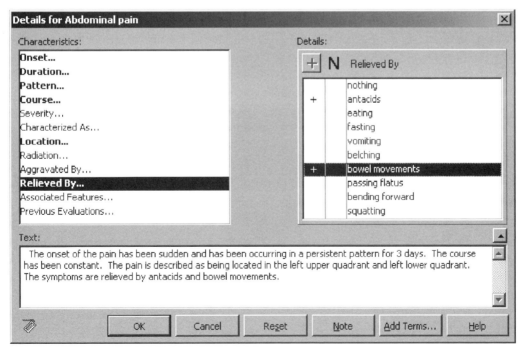

FIGURE 5.3

Notes

Free form note tools are another form of EMR. Information, such as transcription and notes, entered by the doctor may not offer the same access and search capabilities as a knowledgebase or a form. Knowledgebases and forms consist of discrete data items that have a specific definition. In a free form note, the significance of information is driven by the context. For example, you can electronically search knowledgebase or forms EMR data item search to compile a list of your patients with diabetes. If you search a large number of notes for the word "diabetes," then you will end up with a list of patients that have the word diabetes in their note, but do not necessarily have disease (Ex. A relative has diabetes.)

Several hybrid systems include a mix of these different EMR models.

You should consider the types of EMR in your short list to insure that you have a variety of structures or that you exclude product types that will not meet your needs. For example, if your doctors do not want to chart at time of service than you may want to focus on note and document management based EMRs. If you are interested in performing computer assisted analyses of your clinical data, then you need to insure that the EMR will store and manage the specific information entered.

MANAGEABLE LIST OF CANDIDATES

Ideally, you want a manageable number of products to start the detailed review process. Too many potential candidates will be difficult to keep track of, and too few product options may result in a limited view of your choices. ***TIP***: Keep your short-list to 3–4 products. Many on the initial lists could be eliminated based on the paring strategy.

Using the cataloging and elimination strategies in this chapter, you should feel confident that the products on your short-list are viable candidates worthy of your detailed review.

Reviewing Products for Your Practice

Ideally, your EMR product reviews can be completed within 2 months. Some practices stretch out the process for months. Unfortunately, the longer process can risk derailing your efforts and cause fatigue within your entire review team. Other risks of extended reviews include:

Additional product releases may require updates, and, in some cases, force a reexamination of the original review.

Over time, you may forget product specifics. Indeed, some vendors jockey for the last demonstration of the product to make the most lasting impression.

Physicians and staff may lose interest in a project that drags on.

EMR REVIEW PREPARATIONS

Initially, the practice should select who will review the EMR products. A comprehensive EMR review requires technical, clinical, operational, and user interface analysis. In addition to viewing the demonstration, the reviewer(s) needs to analyze what is being done and how the product works. In some cases, practices use outside consultants to review the EMR products. If the review will be performed by internal resources, you should appoint a small review team to look at the products and measure them against your evaluation list. The team should include a strong clinical person who understands charting needs as well as an operational person who understands current patient service and workflow issues. If possible, the team should also include a person knowledgeable in computer applications.

The review team should meet before any demonstrations to review the evaluation list and discuss what the practice needs. The team members should discuss what they are looking for in each item as well as the relative importance of each one. The team should examine some sample screen shots (see some examples later in this chapter) and other materials on each product to gain a general understanding of what they will be looking at. Some vendors even have demonstration disks or websites that your team can view. **TIP:** All of the reviewers should take advantage of CDs and Web sites to become familiar with the products to be reviewed in detail. The initial effort will help you make the best use of your detailed analysis.

To complete the evaluation, you should have a clear strategy for the vendor demonstration. Many vendors want to show you their highlights, but may avoid getting into the details of their product. You should notify the vendor upfront on the general areas that you want to discuss and see demonstrated. For example, you can tell them the key clinical areas that you want to review as well as the ordering system, workflow, prescriptions and other items. **TIP**: Give them actual clinical examples and see how the product performs under each scenario.

You can utilize several different methods to help the vendor set up for the demo:

Limited information—Many practices give no information or demonstration requirements to the vendor. Unfortunately, this gives the vendor an out for any items that the product cannot handle. If you give the vendor guidelines upfront, you can use the evaluation list to challenge the vendor on missing capabilities. For example, if you don't challenge the vendor, the vendor may avoid showing you how the system functions with a certain subspecialty. If you give vendors information to focus the demonstration, and they cannot address your scenario, then the product may not be appropriate, and/or their sales process is not designed to address your needs. **ALERT:** If the product cannot be made to look good in a demonstration, then you should be concerned with what will happen when you try to install the EMR.

Evaluation list—Giving the vendor your evaluation list is your choice. If you give the vendor the evaluation list, the salesperson may fill out the list for you and challenge your analysis. If you do not give the vendor the list, the vendor may claim that they are not prepared for your question or require more resources. Either way, you or your consultant should score the product independently for each evaluation criteria. **TIP**: You are welcome to use the vendor evaluation as a reference, but you should assign your own scores to each item. For example, the vendor may use a task to track a clinical requirement and tasks may not be visible from the patient record when you open the chart. Such a design would complicate identifying important clinical issues for a patient.

Scenario list—Consider sharing a scenario list with the vendor instead of your evaluation list. The scenario list itemizes various processes or activities that demonstrate the flow of patients in your practice. The scenario may cover the handling of patients at the front desk and the handoff to the clinical area. In the clinical area, the scenario may cover the collaboration of nurses and doctors as well as patients receiving various tests and ancillary services. The purpose of the scenario is to walk through a familiar process on the EMR. You'd get a feel for the use of the clinical content and EMR flow. A sample scenario list follows:

- Demonstrate How the Doctor Knows a Patient is Waiting
- Review Initial Patient Information
  — Patient Summary Screen
  — Outstanding Clinical Services (Ex. Tests and Immunizations)
  — Records for a Previous Visit
- Chart Visit
  — Document Chief Complaint
  — Record Previous Medications and Conditions
  — Note Information Available for a Primary Care Visit
    ▪ Record Subjective Primary Care Findings
    ▪ Record Objective Primary Care Findings
    ▪ Document Primary Care Analysis
  — Demonstrate the Information Available for a Cardiology Visit
    ▪ Record Subjective Cardiology Findings
    ▪ Record Objective Cardiology Findings
    ▪ Document Cardiology Analysis
- Complete Clinical Visit
  — Record Plan
    ▪ Lab Orders
    ▪ Diagnostic Study
    ▪ Treatments
    ▪ Prescriptions
    ▪ Recalls
  — Record Charge Information
    ▪ Discuss Support for E&M Codes
- Distribute Patient Education Information
- Sign Chart Note

Be sure to explain to the vendor the importance of the demonstration structure. You should consider telling the vendor how you chose them for a detailed analysis and emphasize the seriousness of your process. The vendor will know that it's on a short list and involved in a serious selection process. In some cases, vendors will be inspired to prepare for your practice and conduct a productive demonstration. Some vendors will not prepare for the demonstration regardless of the amount of information you provide. Failure to prepare under your guidelines should raise a red flag on the capabilities of the product and/or vendor.

EMR SCREEN SAMPLES

Conducting the review and gathering information on your evaluation items requires some familiarity with general screen contents as well as the product your are reviewing. This section presents selected sample screens and general comments on items you should look for. The screen samples are not an endorsement of any particular product; they are used for illustration purposes only.

Patient Summary Screen—The patient summary screen displays a list of the pertinent documents and key information that is stored in the EMR. The user should be able to access the detailed information from the patient summary screen. Verify that you can access the key care information that you need for a patient. For example, a pediatric practice needs to access pending immunization or checkup information while an orthopaedic practice may need to access outstanding orders and incoming MRI results. Some products allow the practice or each user to select the specific information that will be displayed on their patient summary screen. Thereby, nurses can see key information and vitals, while doctors may be more interested in presented results and continuity of care issues. The following sample patient summary is from the MISYS EMR (Figure 6.1).

FIGURE 6.1

Workflow Screen—The workflow screen displays pending work items as well as the status of patients in the office. The list of current patient appointments should directly access the appropriate patient chart. The outstanding to-do's should support more extensive information on the patient issue. Depending on your practice size, you may want to view workflow screens for individual people, doctors, and/or practice units (Ex. Locations, pods, modality, department.) The workflow screen is a key component of the EMR since your staff and doctors will be constantly referencing the screen to identify the next patient or issue to work on. Note that some EMRs only focus on doctors in their workflow screens. The following sample workflow screen is from NextGen EMR (Figure 6.2).

FIGURE 6.2

Patient Information Entry—Patient information entry screens allow patients to enter information that can be posted to the EMR. Practices should be able to customize the patient information entry screen to meet their specific needs. Some EMR products have self contained patient entry screen while other EMRs work with an Internet application to accept information into the EMR. Typically, the information entered by the patient is accepted into the EMR by an authorized user. Patient information entry is an important tool to improve efficiency since it allows the practice to accept information from the patient without having to reenter information from the patient information and intake sheet. This feature can also speed up the doctor since they do not have to dictate the patient information that has been accepted into the EMR record. The following sample patient information entry screen is from Allscripts Healthmatics EMR (Figure 6.3):

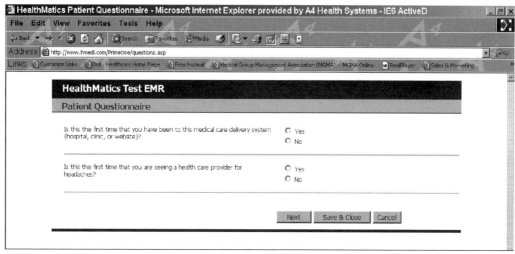

FIGURE 6.3

Message/To-Do Screen—The message/to do screen is used to enter information on outstanding items for patients. The to-do's may be associated with a document (e.g., a radiology study) that triggered the to-do. To-do's may be assigned to specific resources or groups of resources (e.g., nurses). Some EMRs consider the messages as part of the patient's medical record, while other EMRs exclude messages from the patient medical record. A few EMRs allow you to optionally accept selected messages as part of the patient record. The role of messages and their relationship to the patient's record can have a big impact on workflow. For example, if the EMR optionally accepts the messages into the patient record, then you need a specific standard and protocol as well as disciplined staff to properly maintain the patient EMR records. The following Message/to-do screen is from the NextGen EMR (Figure 6.4).

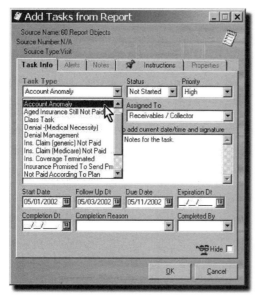

FIGURE 6.4

Clinical Charting—Charting of patient care at time of service is the key to more effective E&M coding, as well as the elimination of transcription. The charting screen should support most of the information that you need to record directly as well as offer the ability to enter a note for information that is not accommodated by the EMR. Make sure that you understand the inclusion and implementation issues of the clinical content for the EMR product. Some vendors sell a defined set of tools to address selected clinical areas, while other vendors provide access to a library where their users can share clinical content. A brief test of clinical charting should be conducted as part of your evaluation. Ideally, you should take a sample note and review the charting process for the note. Make sure that you review the actual note that is produced by the EMR and compare their note to your sample. You should also verify the document production and distribution (Ex. To PCPs, Case Managers) mechanism for clinical information to internal and external parties. The following sample clinical charting screen is from MISYS EMR (Figure 6.5).

FIGURE 6.5

Image Review Screen—Practices accumulate large numbers of images in the EMR. Images may come from scanning of the patient's paper record as well as incoming documents and faxes. The review screen allows the user to select images from a list of patient-related images. Images may be identified by a document type and a description. The EMR should provide viewing options as well as the ability to note issues and items on the image. The following sample image review screen is from SRS (Figure 6.6).

Prescription Screen—Prescription screens are used to record patient medications and produce the appropriate script for the pharmacy. The prescription is automatically entered in a medications' log, as well the patient chart note for that date of service. As a practical matter, the EMR should allow you to enter and track medications from other doctors as well as over the counter drugs being used by the patient. The prescription screen should facilitate the handling and approval of refill requests. The following prescription sample screen is from the Allscripts Healthmatics EMR (Figure 6.7).

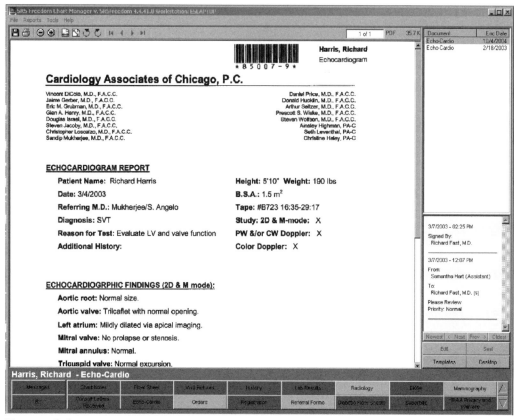

FIGURE 6.6

FIGURE 6.7

Lab Order Screen—This screen accepts information on lab orders and is used to manage the lab test and track the review of results. Lab orders should be managed for lab tests done by the practice as well as lab tests performed by outside parties. Lab modules should also offer a flow sheet view of lab results and a graphing option. The following sample lab order screen is from Allscripts Healthmatics EMR (Figure 6.8).

FIGURE 6.8

Diagnostic Testing Order—Diagnostic tests are entered as part of a patient treatment plan. The EMR should track the diagnostic test through the receipt and review of results. Diagnostic tests may be ordered for recurring issues and patient monitoring. The EMR should monitor tests with a future date as part of a treatment plan. For example, the doctor may want the patient to return with a test in 3 months. Diagnostic tests may be performed by the practice or an outside party. The following sample diagnostic test screen is from MISYS EMR (Figure 6.9).

EMR DEMONSTRATION

The product demonstration has a number of conflicting objectives. You want to quickly review the product, but you also want to get detailed information. The participants will want to see how the product would work in a clinical setting, and everyone wants to pose various permutations. Ideally, you need at least 2–4 hours to go through the basic operation of the EMR as well as get your questions answered. Based on the number of

FIGURE 6.9

specialties, complexity of the practice and number of participants, you may be lucky to get the demonstration done in a day.

At the start of the demonstration, some vendors like to talk about the superiority of their company. They may discuss the company's history, number of employees, revenue growth and client base. Although this is useful information, the introduction should only consume a few minutes. Some vendors have a canned demonstration and others will ask you what you want to see. In the event that the vendor takes too long talking about their company, feel free to ask them to move onto the demonstration.

You should consider having the vendor run through a patient visit without interruption. Although you will be tempted to ask questions, the evaluation team should just sit back and get a look at the flow of the product. **TIP**: Remember to take advantage of their CDs or Web site to prepare for the demonstration. In some cases, practices may perceive that the system is slow and hard to use since they never saw the optimal flow and use of the system during the demonstration. **CAUTION**: If you let the vendor drive the product run through, you could end up with an impractical "sunny day" scenario. In order to get the most out of you demonstration, the vendor should be provided with a scenario and note that represents a real visit to your practice. **TIP**: After the uninterrupted run-through, have the vendor repeat the demonstration more slowly and stop at each key point in which you need a clarification or additional information. The initial run through prepares you for a more detailed discussion of the product in the second viewing of the process.

Using your evaluation list, you should methodically grade each item against the vendor demonstration (see Chapter 4—Compiling a Practice Focused Evaluation List). As you work through the evaluation, make a note for each item that satisfies your evaluation list. Comment on any problems you uncover as well as any particularly effective or impressive features you see.

The note will help participants remember the details of the demonstration. The note is also useful to refute challenges from vendors, doctors and staff, if and when, you discuss any problems. For example, you may award a "1" for a product that had a workaround that was difficult to use, or for an item that would require an excessive amount of work. Ideally, each staff member who is on the review team should take his own notes. The various areas of expertise will assure that your get a comprehensive view of how the product would work. For example, a vendor may suggest using a clinical note to track surgery scheduling, but the surgery scheduler may notice that the note would be manually copied when the surgery is assigned a schedule slot.

In the course of the review, make sure you work through each evaluation item. As you analyze the product, insure that you understand how the product meets the requirements for these issues:

Limited Data—Too often, a vendor conducts a demonstration that does not contain the information of setups to address your questions and issues. Demonstration databases that are not realistic, setups for a different kind of practice, missing clinical content for your area of medicine, and inappropriate examples do not provide an effective and adequate view of the product. This limitation indicates a failure on the part of the vendor to prepare for your practice. *TIP*: If the vendor does not have the demonstration set up to address your issues, evaluate the product on what you see, and not what the vendor claims.

Product Customization—In the event that the vendor offers to customize the product to meet your requirements, you should seriously consider whether any credit should be given for the requirement. Some vendors admittedly are developing their product by adding new features requested by other users. But not all features require the same level of effort. For example, an allergy shot chart is easier to add to an EMR than a workflow management tool. Promises of customization may get a note, but deserve a score of "0." However, you should note any customization commitments for additional analysis if you choose the product. *TIP*: Include the customization requirement in your contract with the vendor.

Upcoming Enhancement—In some cases, the evaluation criteria will be addressed in a forthcoming release by the vendor. You should make a note of the release containing the feature. However, the evaluation should be based on the current capability of the product. *TIP:* Similar to customization, upcoming enhancements could be included in your contract.

Qualify Workarounds—In some cases, the EMR will not be able to do what you are asking and the vendor will suggest a workaround using another feature or more general capability. For example, the vendor may suggest "to-do's" or a note to track pending procedure orders. However, the EMR may lack a connection between the pending order and the supporting note. You would have to monitor the procedure order in the medical record as well as the "to do." Getting from the note to the procedure task could be complicated. In many cases, the workarounds may not be practical to deal with your issues. If the workaround is obscure or does not meet the requirement, you should not give full credit. If you understand and can live with the workaround, credit the vendor accordingly.

Complexity of Features—When the vendor is demonstrating a feature, note how easy the vendor can access the information or demonstrate the capability. If the vendor makes it look difficult or explains the problems with the feature, then you should be concerned with how easy the product will be. For example, the vendor may have to go to 3 or more screens to document a basic issue on your evaluation list. In situations where the product looks difficult, you may want to verify your impression with another viewing of the process. If the product meets the requirement in a complex and difficult matter, you should not award full credit for the criteria.

Comparable Vendor Examples—Solicit comparable practice examples from each vendor. You may solicit these examples indirectly by asking how similar practices deal with one of your key issues. For example, you may ask "show us how primary care practices track immunization shots with the EMR" or "how does the doctor notify the surgery scheduler of a patient treatment need." The lack of examples may indicate that the product cannot handle your requirement or the vendor lacks comparable practice clients.

Verbal Explanations—Sometimes vendors verbally explain how the product works but cannot demonstrate the capability. ***ALERT:*** In some cases, you are viewing screen shots of the EMR and are not even seeing the actual product in use. Common excuses are that the vendor does not have the current version of the software or lacks the clinical content for your specialty. ***ALERT:*** Verbal explanations are a red flag. You should request another demo with the correct version or base the evaluation score on the capability you observed through the software.

Defer to the PMS—Some EMR vendors suggest that certain features should be handled by the PMS. For example, a vendor with an EMR that lacks a patient flow feature may suggest that the patient be tracked through the PMS. However, you are evaluating the issue as part of your EMR selection process and you should verify that you have a workable EMR solution. For example, the recall information may be recorded in the clinical note but not be accessible to the appointment scheduling module when a patient is scheduled for an appointment. Indeed, one vendor suggested giving the patient a post-it note to give to the check-out person for appointment scheduling. Even if your PMS has a certain feature, the PMS should not affect your EMR evaluation—or all of the reviewed EMRs get credit for your PMS' capabilities, which doesn't make sense.

Outstanding Issue—In some cases, the vendor may not have any answer for your evaluation item. The vendor will promise to get back to you. The evaluation items should be scored without the explanation and issue noted. ***CAUTION:*** In some cases, vendors just do not have an answer to your requirement but want to stay competitive. In other cases, you may receive promises but never get an answer.

When you have completed going through the evaluation list, review the items to insure that all of the evaluation items have been scored. Outstanding issues may result in a change to your evaluation but you should verify that all of the issues have been discussed.

Before completing the demonstration and evaluation session, be sure to cover the following additional issues:

Upcoming Releases and Enhancements—The vendor should supply information on upcoming releases and enhancements. For example, you may request a list of the enhancements in the last release as well as enhancements in the next release. You may need specific feedback on enhancements that meet some of the evaluation list items. Such explanations should be in writing and may be included in your contract. For example, a vendor may be adding a drawing tool to the EMR but you will need to know what the drawing tool will offer and how it would work with the image module.

Support Strategy—Have the vendor explain its support strategy. You need to understand how it will address hardware and software issues. Note the support hours and the expected level of expertise in the practice. For example, some EMR vendors limit support contact to a practice employee who has passed a vendor test. A number of EMR vendors have limited support hours or offer a questionable off-hours support strategy. The support strategy should be reviewed against your own support plan and approach. For example, if your practice has a dedicated EMR support person, you will want access to someone who is capable of supporting your EMR point-person. Practices have been frustrated with vendor support staff less knowledgeable about the EMR that the practice employee making the call. Ideally, the vendor should offer contact with a high-level person to insure you get the appropriate support.

Implementation Strategy—The practice should understand how the vendor intends to implement the EMR. In addition to its standard methodology, you should understand how the vendor will deal with your practice's issues. For example, you should be able to discuss how the EMR vendor works with your hardware vendor. Similarly, you need to verify that the vendor can support an implementation strategy that fits your needs. Many vendors require practice staff for management and implementation efforts that should be clearly understood by the practice. Some vendors only offer training services during regular business hours. Thereby, you can prepare your doctors and staff for the time and effort needed to support the implementation process. The vendor should have a clear plan for working with a practice of your size and complexity. For example, an implementation strategy that requires training at the vendor site for all staff may not work if the vendor training facility is far away. **CAUTION**: Some EMR vendors assume that the practice handles hardware, training and even software installation. By understanding your implementation obligations for each vendor, you will avoid surprises later. Knowing your implementation responsibilities could affect the cost of a system. For example, some vendors include implementation of hardware in their installation fees. Your practice would incur additional expenses with another product that would require more resources and costs.

Training Options and Program—You should discuss the various training options (e.g., Train-the-Trainer and direct-user training) offered by the vendor. You should understand the type of training offered and the ability of the vendor to train the people on your staff. Most vendors offer a single set of classes that may not allow you to focus your program on the training needs of your various staffers. You should also review the materials offered by the vendor that can be used to train and support your staff. A number of vendors have developed Web based training programs and CDs that are an integral part of their training services. These options provide flexibility for your practice, but require that each employee have the time and resources to access and participate in the training program. **TIP**: Be certain that you can use the training materials to develop your own.

Online Help and Documentation—You should review samples of online help and printed documentation. Be especially careful to determine the level and quality of the documentation. Some vendors lack sufficient documentation to explain their product. Specialty-specific clinical templates may lack any documentation. **ALERT**: Poor documentation may inhibit your ability to justify an error in the EMR.

At the end of the demonstration, the vendor will typically ask how the product measures up to what you are looking for. You can provide as much information as you wish but you should avoid getting involved in an informal exchange of information outside of the formal review process. Upon hearing of a problem, some vendors may verbally explain the EMR features that address the problem. You are welcome to reopen the demo, but you should not change your evaluation, unless you actually see the solution work.

After the demonstration, call the review team together to compare notes—without the vendor present. **TIP**: Schedule the meeting as soon as possible after the demo. A delay of a few days may undermine your final evaluation. The team should review each evaluation item and develop a consensus evaluation by line item. The consensus evaluation should be the basis for making your final decision and selection.

REQUEST FOR PROPOSAL

A request for proposal (RFP) solicits an EMR product that meets the specifications from your evaluation list. The RFP kicks off the formal EMR selection process. The RFP is typically sent to a selection of EMR vendors to qualify the vendor for further consideration. In some cases, you send the RFP to every vendor. In other cases, the vendor must be prequalified before it gets the RFP. A number of larger companies require the use of RFPs for major purchases. For example, practices that are units of a publicly held corporation may require the use of an RFP. ***TIP***: Most private practices do not use the RFP process.

> ***TIP***: To save you time, and to focus on getting vendors to respond, determine viable vendors for your practice (see Chapter 5—Selecting Products to Review) and send the RFP to these vendors. Otherwise, you may spend time working with and reviewing vendor proposals that have no chance of winning your business.

Be aware that your RFP could scare off vendors. For example, a large practice that seeks an inexpensive product typically used in solo practices may seem illegitimate to vendors.

Regardless of the number of vendors you select, some will not respond to your RFP. To increase your change of getting a response, send RFPs to at least 5 vendors. Certainly limit your RFP distribution to 10–15 vendors.

Begin the RFP by introducing your organization. Describe the number of employees and locations as well as the services you offer. The RFP will continue with an explanation of the selection and evaluation process. The composition of the evaluation team and schedule for the evaluation and implementation process may be included. The RFP articulates the scoring and review process as well as the proposed contract terms and, in some cases, a project plan. The scoring plan will include the specific scoring scales as well as how the scores will be awarded. For example, the RFP may include the weight item for each evaluation list entry as well as the relative value of the evaluation list, implementation plan, support strategy and price in making the final decision.

RFPs can vary widely in length, from a few pages to 50 or more. To increase your chance of getting a response from a vendor, make your RFP concise and direct. Ten to 20 pages should be sufficient for most practices. Don't spend more than a page or two describing your organization, and devote the bulk of the rest of the RFP to your evaluation criteria. The scoring process and contract terms should only be included if your practice or parent organization requires this information in its RFPs.

The RFP may include the evaluation list and, in some cases, detailed information on specific capabilities and features. For example, the RFP may require an interface with a selected PMS system and specify interface data. The RFP also includes information to support the creation of a cost proposal for the EMR purchase. For example, the RFP may list the sites, number of employees by type and volume of business.

Vendors are expected to indicate their ability to meet the features and requirements as well as to submit a cost proposal for the requested products and services. Vendors are expected to comment on any contract terms and conditions that may be a problem for them. As a practical matter, know that vendors do not necessarily always provide the information you seek.

EMR vendors are not going to invest a significant amount of time responding to an RFP that will eliminate their product from further consideration. Some vendors will not respond to RFPs at all since they have other potential customers. Some vendors see the RFP as an opportunity to get their foot in the door of a practice and answer all of your questions in a skewed, positive light.

Although RFPs may have problems, they allow the practice to screen a large number of vendors at a relatively low cost. The vendors who respond to the RFP are considered interested and those vendors who did not respond can be easily eliminated.

After receiving the responses from the vendors, the practice will compile the results to compare vendor proposals. The RFP responses will be compiled and evaluated in much the same way information is compiled from the demo results.

Based on a review of the responses, a select number of vendors will be invited to demonstrate the product for the selection team. This demonstration should be managed using the same strategies described above.

For many practices, an RFP will not necessarily help you advance the EMR project. The results must be verified through your own demonstration. However, the RFP process may be useful, if not required, by larger organizations that may need to engage in an open-selection process.

CHECKING REFERENCES

Reference checking is complicated by the vendor's involvement. References from the vendor may be useful, but keep in mind their references are probably practices that are happy with the system. Ideally, you should seek out references through your own networks and resources. You may call practices you have working relationships with, as well as associations that you may be familiar with. **TIP**: Call the references provided by the vendor and ask the references for other practices they know that use the product. If they mention ones that don't appear on the vendor's list, be sure you contact these practices.

Talk with at least one and preferably two people in the practice. For example, the clinical manager and a doctor may speak with you. The actual reference check should be conducted at a scheduled time and cover:

> **Practice Description**—You should exchange information on your practices. You should get information on size, specialty and clinical focus. For example, practice workflow may not be as important to a smaller practice. You should discuss their operation, patient service style and services offered. You should also verify the use of the EMR in light of your expectations. For example, a reference site may be using the PMS portion, but may be working on installing the EMR.

The interaction between the EMR and PMS should be discussed. You want to verify the viability of connecting your PMS with the reviewed EMR.

EMR Process—Discuss their selection process and implementation experience. Get the names of key vendor players and comments on their performance. You should seek out the identity of knowledgeable support staff, project managers and other vendor staff. You'll identify key vendor staff that can help your EMR effort. You may also get a whiff of any employee turnover problems within the vendor, which can tell you something.

EMR Use—You should discuss the use of the EMR in the practice. Ask about information on workflow changes, successes and failures as well as strategies used to succeed. Gather information on charting, workflow and paper medical records. Make sure you follow-up on any of your concerns and special issues. Current users of the EMR may have more practical advice and solutions than the vendor trainers and support staff.

A sample form for reference checking and site visits is contained at the end of this chapter.

CONDUCTING SITE VISITS

Site visits are useful to review an actual implementation of the EMR, as well as familiarizing yourself with the potential of the EMR. Site visits are expensive due to the loss of office time, and in some cases, travel expenses. However, site visits allow you to see the product in action, and to interact with someone who has gone through the process.

Before committing to a site visit, you should conduct an interview similar to a reference check. Make sure that the practice is a comparable operation. Ideally, the practice should be of similar size and clinical focus to yours. You should also verify the use of the EMR in light of your expectations. For example, an office that is not paperless may not be a good site visit for a practice that wants a paperless medical record.

Make sure you talk about your practice's situation and objectives. You may also discuss their selection process, implementation experience and the objectives of your visit. You should explain the size of your site visit team and verify that the activities that your want to see will be taking place while you're there. For example, avoid a day when few patients are scheduled and the doctors are in surgery.

Your site visit team should consist of at least one clinician and one operations person. The site visit should allow the team to view the current operation and use of the EMR. The visit should include viewing the use of the EMR during a patient visit, as well as how information flows in the office. Ideally, your team should run through the entire operation and view all areas where the EMR is in use.

After each site visit, your entire EMR evaluation team should meet to discuss the findings and observations of the site visit team. The key successes and problems should be noted as well as strategies that the practice should use in its continuing EMR efforts, including possible additional site visits.

EMR REFERENCE CHECK/SITE VISIT QUESTIONNAIRE

Practice Name: _____ Phone: _____

Type: _____

Number of: Doctors: _____ Staff: _____ Locations: _____

Contact: _____ Position: _____

What were 3 key compelling reasons that the practice bought the product?

1.

2.

3.

What were 3 areas where the product has exceeded the practice's expectations?

1.

2.

3.

Cite 3 areas where the product has not met your practice's expectations.

1.

2.

3.

Evaluate the following vendor services:

Implementation: ❑ Poor   ❑ Average   ❑ Good   ❑ Outstanding

Why? _____

_____

Training: ❑ Poor   ❑ Average   ❑ Good   ❑ Outstanding

Why? _____

_____

Continuing Support: ❑ Poor   ❑ Average   ❑ Good   ❑ Outstanding

Why? _____

_____

Date product was used as the primary source of your medical record information: _____

Was the date above: ❏ Before   ❏ On   ❏ After the expected activation date?

Why?   _____

_____

Has the practice eliminated paper medical records?   ❏ Yes   ❏ No

If yes, how long did it take to eliminate paper medical records and what were the key issues/problems you ran into:

_____

_____

If no, what are the reasons that you still use paper medical records:

_____

_____

In what ways is the EMR superior to paper medical charts?

1.

2.

3.

In what ways is the current EMR not as good as paper medical charts?

1.

2.

3.

What were the key strategies used to transition the doctors to the EMR?

1.

2.

3.

If you could go back through the implementation of the EMR, what would you change?

_____

_____

_____

What advice do you have for our practice in implementing the EMR product?

_____

_____

_____

Please rate the effect of the new EMR in the following areas:

Patient Service	❏ Less Effective	❏ Same	❏ Improved
Clinical Workflow	❏ Less Effective	❏ Same	❏ Improved
Staff Productivity	❏ Less Effective	❏ Same	❏ Improved
Doctor Productivity	❏ Less Effective	❏ Same	❏ Improved
Record Accuracy	❏ Less Effective	❏ Same	❏ Improved

How long did it take before things calmed down (non-chaotic) after EMR implementation? _____

Why? _____

_____

What specific items were done to help speed this process? _____

_____

Making a
Final Decision

The final selection of the EMR is rarely a slam dunk proposition. If that were the case, far fewer that 400 different options would be offered in the marketplace. Typically, the EMR decision is mostly a choice between closely matched product options.

To make a final decision, you need to focus on the key differences between the products based on the information you have compiled. If you try to rationalize 100 or more items, then you may have difficulty working through the analysis.

Your final decisions should be based on an analysis of your product evaluation as well as a clear understanding of the costs of each EMR.

SUMMARIZING THE EVALUATION

Compiling the information from your evaluation into a meaningful summary is a challenge. You could have hundreds of data points and many comments. You need to create an easy to understand metric from a complex set of information. Considering the detailed evaluation backs up the summary, you can simplify the comparison as follows:

Eliminate Criteria When all Products Met the Standard—To highlight the differences between the products, you could ignore items where all of the products met the requirement. For example, if all of the EMR products have interfaces with your PMS, then the evaluation criteria could be ignored. Items where product scores differ would not be eliminated. Eliminating these criteria would highlight the quantitative difference between the products. For example, say, three products scored between 200 and 220 in total based on the evaluation effort. If 80 points for each product represented meeting the same exact features, then the difference in scores is actually 120 to 140. The 20-point difference is then more significant as a percentage of the total score.

Categorize Results—Categorizing results helps you focus on areas where the products differ. The total score could obscure issues that may be important for you. For example, serious deficiencies in workflow may be offset by a good training program. The results can be categorized using the categories from your evaluation list. You may compile summary scores for technology, HIPAA support, workflow, interfaces, clinical content, patient order management, patient service, training, reporting, cost and support.

Weighted Scores—A weighted score is calculated by multiplying the evaluation score by an importance factor. You may assign importance factors to each evaluation item or to the category. For example, you may use a weighting factor of 3 for critical requirements, 2 for general items and 1 for nice-to-have features. The weighted scores ensures that a less important requirement does not offset a more important item. For example, you may assign a low weight to PMS interface and a high weight to workflow capabilities.

Occurrence Summaries—Occurrence summaries are counts of the number of scores received by each product in each scoring category (e.g., 10–0s, 21–1s, 57–2s, and 26–3s). The occurrence summary quantitatively presents the number of deficiencies and does not shield problems with outstanding scores in other areas. For example, missing lab order features will not be offset by outstanding workflow features. Occurrence summaries will help you identify the product that met the most requirements.

These various scoring methods are not mutually exclusive. You may calculate and consider all of these measures in making your final decision.

HARDWARE PROVISIONING

In a typical EMR purchase, hardware represents 20%-40% of the EMR cost. EMR implementations frequently result in massive changes to the current practice technology base. You may have some existing hardware that you intend to use with the system but you will **probably not have the number of workstations needed** to support an EMR. Most practices will need to buy the main EMR computer server, additional workstations, tablet devices, scanners and a whole host of equipment and system licenses. Indeed, you may have to replace substantial portions of your technology infrastructure to handle the EMR.

How these changes are implemented and who is responsible for these changes will be part of your final decision process. Excluding all other issues (including cost), you would prefer to have a single vendor and point of responsibility. However, hardware provisioning varies widely among EMR vendors. Some EMR vendors sell all of the hardware you need directly, while other EMR vendors have a preferred hardware vendor. Several EMR vendors do not sell any hardware. Some EMR vendors are not competitive on price, and many vendors do not want to accept responsibility for your existing hardware.

Depending on your situation, the practice should decide from whom the hardware will be purchased. As a practical matter, you have three options: (1) Buy all hardware from the EMR vendor, (2) buy all hardware from another source (e.g., local systems integrator) or (3) purchase the server from the EMR vendor and other hardware from other sources.

If you have a current hardware supplier, you may be tempted to buy equipment from it. Since your existing vendor knows your system, the vendor will be able to more effectively analyze the changes that are needed. **ALERT:** However, your existing vendor may lack experience with the EMR product. Nonetheless, some practices have gone to the expense of keeping their local supplier involved in the EMR project. Continuing involvement may include paying the local vendor to get trained on the setup of the EMR and your new hardware as well as serving as a technical advisor to the practice. Under this arrangement, you maintain a local resource that may be able to more quickly respond to problems and more easily keep track of continuing advancements for your system. An added benefit of using the local vendor is that the local resource can serve as a sounding board for any technical issues raised or specified by your EMR vendor. For example, you EMR vendor may sell one brand of hardware since they get the best deal, but another hardware vendor may have better support in your local area. Similarly, the EMR vendor may have limited experience with high availability systems that you may choose to use. **CAUTION**: If you change hardware vendors or use the EMR vendor for your hardware, you will have to pay the new vendor to learn your system.

Some EMR vendors have working relationships with select hardware vendors. Depending on volume, the EMR vendor may or may not have much influence with the hardware vendor. In some cases, the hardware vendor may not have a good support system in your area and you may end up with hardware support from a local third party. The EMR hardware vendor may not understand your current hardware system or setup. **CAUTION:** Many hardware vendors may come into your practice and recommend a number of changes. In some cases, the recommendations will not improve your situation, but will bring your system in line with their "standard products." For example, the vendor may prefer a different backup device and software product even though your existing backup system may be adequate or even more widely used. Unfortunately, the "standard products" usually aren't better that the products you have currently installed.

If your practice buys hardware components from a variety of sources, you may encounter problems holding anyone accountable for problems. A variety of vendors can be particularly vexing when you are trying to solve a problem. For example, one practice couldn't get their tablets from one vendor to work with the practice's wireless network from another vendor. All of the tablets had to be replaced. Interestingly, the replacement was not technically necessary, but the two vendors could not agree on a workable solution and strategy. Due to these problems, the project was delayed several months.

Similarly, practices that try to mix and match equipment may have problems getting the entire system to work together.

You could end up paying several vendors to learn each other's products and solve your problems. **CAUTION**: On occasion, the only way to solve a problem is to have a representative from each of the vendors working on the problem together in your facility and billing your account. To avoid such problems, the practice should have an in-house or local advisor to maintain current information on the system and act as the practice's advocate in dealing with the various vendors. For more technical issues, you may even have a more experienced local technical resource to supplement your own staff for more complex problems.

The best strategy is to limit the variables and vendors. If you have a local hardware support group, you may be better off letting it handle your computer network, workstations, tablets, scanners, network infrastructure and installation. Of course, if you have an internal IT support staff, you are in a better position to mix and match hardware sources. **TIP**: Another way to limit issues is to assign support for the EMR server to the EMR vendor. The EMR vendor is responsible for managing the one point in the system where your alternative hardware vendor may lack expertise. The clear line of responsibility will help you keep the vendors accountable for their areas and limit the points of dispute.

The hardware purchase should be supported by the hardware standards from the EMR vendor. In comparing various vendors, you will find that most EMR products use the same basic hardware. However, products may differ in their hardware requirements. For example, some vendors require separate test and production servers, while others may require a separate server for the EMR and a dedicated server for images. A few products can even put the entire EMR setup on a single server. EMR vendors may also require different types of access to your system and control over the various aspects of your installation. For example, some vendors will not provide the passwords to administer their EMR servers. **TIP**: Make sure that the EMR vendor has published hardware specifications that you can rely on to configure the hardware for your specific situation.

Your hardware selection and strategy reflects your tolerance for a system loss. This strategy can affect the cost of a system. Your hardware strategy may include the following.

High-Availability Hardware—High availability hardware includes redundant components that allow the EMR to operate in the event of certain hardware failures. For example, a power supply failure will not affect a system with redundant power supplies. Cluster servers offer an even higher level of availability by providing you with "twin systems" to support the EMR. If a component fails in the main server, the clustered server immediately takes over. Due to continued drops in cost, cluster server setups are available for under $30,000. Additional protection is available by allowing for multiple servers in your network to manage system resources and performance. For example, a network uses an active directory server (ADS) to keep track of what all the users are doing. A problem with the ADS could cause a complete system failure. However, for a relatively modest additional investment, you could add a second ADS to your system. A variety of other components (Ex. Routers, Tablets, Workstations, Scanners) can be protected and backed up according to your tolerance for failure balanced with the cost of the additional protection.

Server Hosting—Your EMR and other servers could be placed with a computer-hosting or co-location organization. The computer-hosting facility typically provides power generators and batteries to avoid problems due to power failures as well as redundant communication lines. The hosting facility will also be secured and include environmental controls for your system. In some cases, the hosting company will provide backup hardware in the event of EMR server failure. Hosting fees would be included in your cost comparison. For example, one vendor may have an arrangement with a hosting facility that is less expensive that the other vendors. **ALERT:** Hosting facilities typically charge a monthly fee and may have usage-based fees. You may also incur additional expenses for communications expenses from the main office (that would have severed as the EMR-server location) to the host site. **TIP:** A number of communication companies that you buy your data lines from may offer co-location services at a discount when you buy a package of services.

ASP (Application Services Provider)—Many EMR products are available through ASPs. ASPs provide the servers to support selected EMR products as well as the hosting facility. The ASP charges are typically based on users and provider-based fees on top of the hosting fees. The ASP strategy will minimize your upfront license cost since the ASP owns the licenses that they rent to your practice. **CAUTION:** ASP offerings vary widely in what is included in the fee and what your practice gets for the fee. For example, some ASP costs do not include training and initial implementation costs. **TIP:** If you choose the ASP option, make sure that you fully understand the "exit" strategy in the event that you switch to another product in the future, or decide to bring the EMR inhouse.

Backup Sites—Some EMR vendors now offer backup sites that could be used in the event of a catastrophic loss of your system. On a periodic basis, you new data is sent to the backup site and posted to an operational version of your database. In the even of a system loss, your users would be switched to the backup site and have access to your data as of the last update. Note that updates could occur with every transaction, every hour, or within any other period you choose.

Backup Servers—Blade servers allow you to quickly replace a defective server with an operational server. Blade servers are less expensive than cluster servers and can be swapped by a trained computer support person.

Hardware issues should be resolved as you work on compiling the EMR cost comparison. As you prepare the cost comparison, you will develop your hardware strategy and sources. The cost comparison will more closely reflect the final purchase costs and strategy.

COMPARING PRODUCT COSTS

Comparing costs of products is intentionally complex. Vendors do not want you to price shop their offering and products. Vendor pricing strategies and service levels vary widely. For example, one vendor quoted 175 hours of implementation support, while a competing vendor quoted almost 400 hours of support. Which vendor was right? Using the same hourly rate, was the 400-hour vendor more expensive?

To compare product costs, you should solicit a proposal based on the specific hardware, software and services needed to implement the EMR. At this point in your process, you should ask for the vendor's best and final quote. Otherwise, you will have to update your analysis each time the vendor updates its proposal. Many vendors calculate the number of users based on classifications of various staff types (e.g., doctors, mid-levels, nurses, technicians and non-clinical users). Other vendors have a single license fee for all users. Either way, the number of users will be an important issue for the vendor. The following information should be presented to the vendor to insure that you will receive an accurate and practical quote for your practice:

Number of Entities—If your practice operates under a number of corporate entities, you may have to pay a license fee for each entity. In some cases, you may also have to pay user fees for each staff person who may access the EMR. For example, if your practice is associated with a therapy group, optical shop or ASC that is a different corporation, you may have to pay additional fees for the second corporation. Additionally, you may have to pay a separate license fee for a staff member who may need to access information for both organizations (e.g., billing office staffers who work on the practice and the ASC).

Physicians and Providers—The number of physicians and providers should include all medical decision-makers. Many vendors will charge full provider licenses for any party that is billing under his own ID. If your practice uses part-time providers, mid-level providers who bill under a doctor's billing number and residents, don't forget these providers in your budget and your negotiations with the vendor. **ALERT:** A number of vendors charge license fees based on the number of providers but only allow for a specific number of users per provider. For example, you may be allowed only 5 users for each provider even though the license states that you are paying per provider. If you have a higher number of users per provider, you could have to pay additional fees.

Clinical Staff—Clinical staff includes technicians, nurses and other parties. These employees will need access to the EMR, and will count in the user total. **TIP**: Clinical staff may also need additional licenses to access the PMS system. Review the PMS access cost because an integrated system may not require such additional PMS licenses.

Other Users—A variety of administrative, billing and front-desk staff will need access to the EMR to interact with clinical staff and access medical records. The front desk staff may flag a patient who is ready for service as well as notify doctors of scanned medical information. Billing staff may access the medical record to support insurance claims and other functions. **TIP**: Ask for lower cost licenses for non-clinical users. Some vendors will do this. Other vendors include all users equally in the licensed user count.

Locations—The number of locations may affect certain hardware and software issues. Some EMR licenses include additional fees for each location. To support remote locations, you may need additional servers and licensed software. For example, some vendors charge a remote scanning license fee for any office that scans documents.

Hardware Specifications—To receive a realistic hardware configuration, you should specify your hardware requirements. The hardware requirements may include redundant components and fail safe options. For example, you may specify an uninterruptible power supply as well as hot swap disk configurations to mitigate the risk of a system stoppage. You may also ask for a full system proposal and a proposal that only includes the EMR server with all other hardware being supplied by your current hardware vendor. Be sure you consider your entire computer network and not just the vendor requirements. For example, you may use the new system backup for the PMS, document server and other systems, including the EMR. Similarly, you may need an additional server to manage the interface between your EMR and PMS.

Interfaces—The list of expected interfaces should be presented to the vendor. You may need interfaces for the PMS, diagnostic equipment and your lab information system. You may also need an interface for exchanges with hospitals and other practices. In addition to the interfaces you need now, you may also want to get information on any additional interfaces you may need. For example, the next time you are buying diagnostic equipment, consider products that are already interfaced with your EMR. Note that interfaces can require additional hardware. For example, the interface between a piece of diagnostic equipment and the EMR may require an additional workstation in the same room with the diagnostic equipment. **CAUTION**: You may need an interface server to manage the interfaces between the EMR and your PMS, or other devices.

Training and Services—You may include information on your training expectations and/or plan. Key items include the number of people to be trained and whether you will use a train-the-trainer plan. If you are comparing a vendor that uses a train-the-trainer approach versus full vendor training, consider any additional costs you may incur for overtime and/or replacement staff for your internal training effort. For example, you may need to hire your own trainer and set up a training facility. **TIP**: Many practices need more training services than the practice or the vendor anticipates. You should set aside some contingency money for additional training efforts. This will ensure you include the full cost of the training in your comparison. You may also include information on the on-site services you expect for the project. For example, you may have three sites that will require an onsite vendor representative on the Go Live date.

In some cases, vendors will present a single price for the system. However, you will need an unbundled price to compare the product with other proposals. In the event that the vendor will not provide a price breakdown, you may be able to break down the fixed price based on costs you have access to. For example, you may be able to get hardware quotes directly from the hardware vendors and back out services based on the vendor's hourly rate.

Once you have received the proposal or quote, you should compare the proposed systems in a table. A sample budget comparison table is included at the end of this chapter. Note that the table includes various components with a space for costs and maintenance fees. The comparison table also includes a space for contingencies. Vendor-specific contingencies may be based on a number of issues including hardware upgrades that may be needed and additional training services for a more complex technology.

The totals cover the acquisition cost and maintenance cost as well as a projected 5-year cost, including maintenance. The 5-year total expense will help you analyze the true cost of each product. For example, some EMR vendors have low license fees, but high maintenance costs. You can add projections for maintenance cost increases, equipment upgrades and replacements and an imputed interest rate to the cost comparison. You should also compute a monthly cost that can be used to analyze return-on-investment (ROI) and the payback from the projected savings and additional revenues.

Compiling the price comparison does require some analysis and creativity. Consider the following issues.

> **Scope**—Each vendor may include different things in its proposals and costs. Vendors have a variety of methods to calculate charges and the scope of services could vary widely among practices. For example, some vendors omit subscription and acquisition costs for clinical content that may be needed from a third-party vendor. Other vendors may propose a basic system that will require a number of additional components and additional investment. In some cases, the vendor strategy may differ from your own. For example, some vendors provide training, but do not provide any advisory or practice management services. **CAUTION**: Additional services could spike your EMR costs. For example, customization of the EMR could represent a substantial cost that is not accounted for. At a minimum, the practice should allow for some contingency funds for customization. Other vendors include training in the base cost of the software license. Some vendors offer training at their offices while others may train at your office. Travel expenses may have to be weighed. Note that travel costs could be based on situations beyond your control. For example, a vendor may assign resources to your practice that is farther from your location that the vendor's nearest office.

Missing Items—If you have an item for one vendor and not others, then you need to determine if the item is needed or not. In some cases, the additional item is a requirement of the particular EMR. For example, some EMRs require a server to run email, while others have email built into their product. In other cases, the vendor has failed to address all you needs. For example, most practices will want a fax server or similar service to avoid scanning incoming faxes into the EMR. *ALERT:* Some vendors may fail to quote a remote terminal services server needed for remote users. If you have many remote users, and are concerned with performance, you may be able to minimize the communication requirements with a Windows terminal server and perhaps a Citrix metaframe.

Cost Basis—Due to a wide variety of vendor strategies and issues, the EMR cost is frequently obscured. Many products are based on standard hardware infrastructures that are comparable. However, you will want to eliminate differences that you would address in any purchase agreement.

> **Better Hardware**—Hardware prices may vary due to more capacity or additional features to protect you from failure. For example, a $30,000 server may provide you a smaller chance of a complete hardware failure than a basic $10,000 server would. Do you consider the $30,000 server more expensive if it offered greater protection? If the hardware differences are due to better equipment then you should normalize the hardware items to the level of products that you expect to buy. For example, fully redundant disks, power supplies and fans should be included for any practice, but a cluster server (where two systems share a common set of storage devices) may be desired by a large practice. Similarly, a very basic workstation proposed by one vendor may be replaced with a better workstation that would be included in all vendor quotes.

> **Comprehensive Quotes**—Some vendors quote basic systems that you would not buy. For example, they may quote undersized hardware and exclude modules that you will need to buy (e.g., lab system interfaces). In some cases, the quote may not include items that depend upon implementation decisions. For example, if you decide to scan the old paper charts, you will need a lot more storage space. To make sure that you have all of the components you will need, verify the quote against your evaluation criteria as well as inventory the interfaces that you will need. In the event that a vendor does not include a component you know you will need, you can add the item to the vendor quote based on other cost information you may have. For example, you could plug in a tablet price based on a quote you can get from a hardware vendor. If the vendor does not include a price for training, you could apply the vendor's training rate against the expected training hours you'll need from the other vendors.

Implementation Services—Implementation services are frequently quoted as a basket of hours to be used by the practice. However, you can find differences between the rates. Rates for services can range from $75-$250/hour depending on the level of staff and vendor rates. Make sure that the basket of hours proposed by the vendor would meet your requirements. If necessary, adjust the basket of hours to conform to your own implementation needs or the standard. Alternatively, you can assign all vendors the same level of hours and use the quoted vendor rate. Contingency allowances can also be used to permit for differences in the services' quote. For example, one vendor included a "reasonable" training program in the cost of the EMR. However, this estimate was based on a much larger number of hours than what was considered necessary. Note that some vendors limit the time when you can use purchased hours. For example, you may need to use the purchased hours within 12 months of the purchase. Make sure that you do not buy more hours than you can reasonably use during the implementation time limit.

Licenses—Using the number of users, providers and other counts, verify that the proposed license will meet your needs. A slight change in your license count could up the cost of the system. For example, some EMRs are licensed by provider, but only allow so many licenses for each provider. If you are above the users-per-provider count, you may have to pay additional fees. Note that you need to get the correct number of licenses in the analysis for each vendor. Otherwise, you could end up with incorrect figures and harm your comparison. For example, practices that use mid-level providers will want to be certain about how such providers are licensed. *TIP:* Some EMR vendors charge mid-level providers the same price as doctors, while others reduced the rate, sometimes even to nothing. Similarly, some vendors require EMR licenses for non-clinical users (Ex. Billers and appointment schedulers) while other vendors charge for each workstation. Thereby, you would have to pay additional fees for workstations that you may place to promote use of the EMR, but could not possibly be in use at once since your employee count is less than your number of workstations.

Functionality—The cost comparison should account for comparable functionality between the products. For example, one EMR vendor may offer an imaging product that allows for extensive indexing of scanned images. Another vendor may offer a more basic scanning product with the EMR, with an optional module that offers advanced indexing. You should include the more advanced scanning module for a more precise comparison.

Support Costs—Support costs are a major component of any EMR purchase. Support costs can range from 15%-33% of the original license cost on an annual basis. Support costs should include annual payments for clinical content, drug databases and other subscription items. Make sure the support costs account for any other adjustments you have made. Additional hardware and licenses could affect support costs. The support costs should be used to calculate a 5 year system cost. Such an analysis will help you determine the true cost of the system when the vendors use different support cost factors.

Discounts—Some vendors will offer a system discount to compel you to buy the product. The offered discount should be included in the cost comparison. The discount line can be updated as you proceed with vendor negotiations. Note that discounts may be available for end-of-period purchases, combined EMR and PMS purchases and previous customers, among other offers.

Modularization of the Product—Vendors use a dizzying array of packaging techniques to sell their systems. Some EMRs are sold as a complete product with few options. Other vendors may sell a prescription module, transcription module and a clinical charting module. **CAUTION**: Some vendors charge for each area of medicine and/or clinical content package. To assure accuracy, verify that your evaluation requirements are covered by the proposed modules. Otherwise, you could be surprised to find out you need an additional module. You should be especially careful for modules that are included in the companion PMS, but not the PMS that you will use with the EMR. For example, an appointment module may be needed to store appointment information in the EMR that is downloaded from your PMS.

Additional Upgrades—Depending on your situation, you should determine what, if any, additional modifications will be needed for the EMR. Upgrades to your existing network, and licensing current software versions may be necessary and should be included in your comparison. For example, one product may require licenses updates or even new workstations while another product may be able to work with the current system. **Warning:** You may need to move to an updated version of the PMS or the "next generation" PMS product to use the "companion" EMR product.

Clinical Content Development—Many EMR products have clinical content for selected specialties and clinical areas. The clinical content may consist of specific templates, system setups, pick lists and other tools to ease the implementation effort. Some vendors include clinical content assistance while others assume that the practice will perform all of the clinical content setup. Vendors may also offer a forum to access the clinical content setups that have been developed by other practices. Depending on your needs and analysis of the clinical content, you may want to allow for an appropriate level of clinical content support. If you are perfectly content with the current clinical content, then you may need minimal support. If you like the product but expect extensive clinical content changes, then you allow for a higher level of assistance. Note that clinical content development and enhancement can add substantial amounts to the cost of your EMR and lengthen your implementation timeline.

The completed cost comparison permits you to measure the incremental costs with the qualitative differences between the products you are considering.

FINAL DECISION

After collecting information on the capabilities of the product, impressions of staff, reference checks and site visits, you will have an extensive body of data that needs to be consolidated into a manageable and easy-to-understand form. The rest of the practice will not be in the position to review all of the data that you have uncovered.

When summarizing information, be concise. Of course, each of your conclusions will be backed up with the more detailed analyses. You may present a minimalist comparison of the products that merely rates features, support, services, references and cost. You may also provide another level of detail that addresses feature categories and/or cost components. In some cases, a ranking of the products in each category will help crystallize your final analysis. *TIP*: Rank the products as first, second and third in cost, support, features and references. Note that you may want to break down features in your summary into general areas, such as system support, workflow and clinical content.

Note that cost is a factor, but not *the* factor. In many cases, dramatic cost differences between products may be attributed to the different capabilities of the product or the target market. In many cases, you can negotiate away differences between comparable EMR products. However, you should seek a product that will work in your practice over a product that may be less expensive, but may require more labor on your part (e.g., clinical content development).

Feel free to try a couple of these summarization methods to identify the one or two top products for your practice. *TIP*: If you end up without a clear winner, don't panic. You may have been lucky enough to identify more than one product that could be successfully installed in your practice. That is you may have one or more good options that could satisfy your needs.

When presented with this situation, many practices will expend a significant amount of time and effort to arrive at the "best" decision. The lack of a "best" decision may result in no decision at all, but to continue to sap the time and resources in the decision-making process. If you cannot choose one option as the "best," then consider yourself fortunate and make a decision. In reality, you need to be careful to not exhaust yourself or the practice in making a decision, and then lack the energy to tackle the hard tasks associated with actual implementation.

Before you go any further, take a reality check. If necessary, call the top 1 or 2 vendors in for another demonstration. You need to be absolutely certain that the product can be effectively implemented and used in your practice. You should be planning the implementation of the product and visualizing the product in your practice to validate your final decision.

The actual presentation of your final recommendation should be carefully staged and prepared. Have your summaries, supporting documentation and list of vendors that you considered. Typically, the recommendation is made during a presentation to the management team, doctors, operations committee or some other group in the practice. The presentation should explain the EMR selection process, discuss options that were explored and then present concise summary information with your recommendation. The presentation should include the go-forward plan for the final decision, necessary negotiations and the implementation process.

As a matter of due diligence, the attendees will ask questions that should require going down a level or two into the details. The object of the meeting should be to pick one or two products and to proceed to the next step.

If you have made your choice or want to continue considering two products, you should feel comfortable if either choice would work for your practice. For the next steps, don't proceed with any product that you could not use.

To build support and enthusiasm for the chosen product or to make the final choice, you should schedule a drop-in day for the remaining vendor(s). The drop-in day is your opportunity to let your doctors and staff, see and touch the product. Don't present any product to the staff that could not realistically be purchased by the practice. The drop-in day should be scheduled to present the system to various groups of doctors and staff. You should schedule four or more sessions that will run through a script (similar to the script used for demonstrations) and allow employees to ask questions. This way, employees have several opportunities to see the product throughout the day and you can rekindle interest in the EMR project as well as jump start everyone on the daunting implementation task ahead.

If you have chosen the product, you can start work on contract negotiations before the drop-in day. If you're down to two final options, seek employee feedback to help you make the ultimate decision. Actively ask for their input. After choosing your EMR product, begin contract negotiations.

After making your final decision, you will hear from doctors and vendors about additional products, updates to products that you considered, and, in some cases, scare tactics to reopen your process. You should be prepared to address these issues in a methodical manner and seek to avoid any serious buyer's remorse. In many cases, the scare tactics are just that. Have enough confidence in your process and the analysis behind your decision to proceed with the selected EMR.

TABLE 7.1

EMR Cost Comparison	PRODUCT 1		PRODUCT 2	
	Cost	Maintenance	Cost	Maintenance
Servers				
EMR Application				
Remote Access				
Imaging				
Backup				
Fax Server				
System Software				
Software				
Wireless Network				
Firewall				
Printers				
Color				
Standard				
Scanners				
Front Desk Page				
Medium Volume				
High Volume				
Workstations/Tablets				
Workstation Upgrades				
Additional Workstations				
Tablets				
Network Upgrades				
Inter-Office				
Intra-Office				
Application Software				
EMR				
Imaging				
PMS Interfaces				
Lab Interfaces				
Diagnostic Interfaces				
Clinical Content				
Installation				

EMR Cost Comparison	PRODUCT 1		PRODUCT 2	
	Cost	Maintenance	Cost	Maintenance
Training				
Monthly Hosting Fees				
Less System Discount				
Totals				
Hardware Contingency				
Software Contingency				
Training Contingency				
Other Contingency				
Total with Contingencies				
5-Year Total Cost				
5-Year Monthly Cost				

Negotiating a Contract

By the time you have decided on a particular system, you may be so exhausted that you are in no position or mood to work your way through page after page of unreadable and less-than understandable contract text. Our first impulse is to rely on the vendor's agreement since "they do this all the time." However, the practice is clearly at a disadvantage since you will be depending on the capabilities and features of the EMR to service all of your patients. Your vendor is only at risk for the dissatisfaction of a single practice.

A contract is an agreement between two parties that establishes the rights and responsibilities of each party. What we think the vendor should do, and stand behind, is frequently very different from what most vendor contracts say. Consider some quick examples:

No Warranty—Many vendors exclude any warranty from your agreement. They will not contractually stand behind their product, services, hardware or software. In the event of a problem with the product, your practice may not have much contractual leverage.

Pay Before they do Anything—Many vendors want 50% of the cost when you sign the contract and another 50% when they drop the boxes of their product on your office floor (or in some cases when they ship the boxes from their plant). So, you have paid all your money out before you even see what's in the box.

Termination Clause—Most vendor contracts empower the vendor to terminate your ability to use the EMR on demand for a whole list of terrible actions including non-payment, letting non-employees see the system, making copies of their materials, moving the system and even buying additional equipment. Of course, the contract does not consider the irreparable harm and severe economic losses that would occur if the practice lost access to the EMR for even a few hours.

You need to be very clear about what you are and are not expecting from the EMR vendor. On the other side, vendors have certain things that they do, and certain things they do not do. Although, you should not buy an EMR or sign a contract with a vendor that you do not trust, you also should ensure that the contract protects your interests and effectively structures your relationship with the EMR vendor.

Your initial contract effort should focus on the business deal and the relationship with the vendor. If you cannot work out the business points, then you should not waste your time trying to decipher the lengthy terms and conditions in the contract documents.

NEGOTIATING BUSINESS POINTS

To make the best use of your time, you need to identify the business relationship and the parties involved in the negotiations. Otherwise, you could spend a lot of time negotiating an agreement that you will never sign since the basic business agreement is not completed or acceptable. For example, you may not be able to get any support for a warranty from the vendor.

Key business points can be significantly affected by the contract terms and other aspects of your agreements with the chosen vendor. The key business points include:

Vendor(s)

One of the more confusing aspects of negotiating contracts for the purchase of an EMR is who you are buying products from. Many EMR vendors are selling components from various vendors that are integral to making their system work. The EMR vendor may be selling software from one company, services from a second company and hardware from a third. In the event of a problem, you could end up in endless expensive discussions between two or more entities. For example, your EMR vendor may sell you software from another vendor to support voice recognition or faxing, but you may have to pay additional fees to the other software vendor to get support for any problems. *TIP:* Some of these situations include a second agreement from the EMR publisher that is presented at the last minute for signing. Make sure that you get copies of all of the agreements and paperwork that you will need to establish the relationship with the vendor and purchase the EMR.

The EMR vendor should take full responsibility for the EMR and the EMR working relationship with the various components regardless of where these components originate. In some cases, the vendor excludes any responsibility for third party software that, unknown to you, is a key component of the product you are buying. For example, your EMR may use a built-in imaging product from a vendor you have not heard of. If the EMR vendor does not take responsibility for working with these key third party components, then you need to identify the other software vendors that you may need to contact in the event of a problem between your EMR and these third party products.

Vendor and Practice Responsibilities

To produce a practical contract and successfully implement the EMR, the practice needs to clearly understand the vendor responsibilities as well as the responsibilities of the practice or other third parties. In most projects, the practice does not get a handle on these issues until the project is well under way. The delay in identifying these responsibilities can lead to a lot of confusion and additional costs.

Unfortunately, many vendors will not let you see their plan until you have purchased their system. Some vendors have extensive lists of tasks in a project management table, while others develop the project plan as you proceed. In most cases, you will need to create your own list of tasks to implement the EMR. Some key issues to understand in the context of the contract follow:

- What vendors are supplying what components?
- Has the EMR vendor verified the components and services purchased from other parties?
- Who will install the hardware?
- Who will install the software on the hardware and verify that the entire system is working?
- What documents will be presented to the practice to explain the hardware configuration?
- What are the training packages and timeframes for the training effort?
- What are the training responsibilities of the vendor and practice?
- What are the project and management responsibilities for the EMR vendor, other vendors and the practice?
- Who will represent the practice in dispute resolution with the EMR vendor?

For more information on managing the EMR implementation, see **Chapter 9—Implementing an EMR**. Make sure you clearly understand how the basic components of the project will be performed and who will be responsible for it.

Price

Many EMR systems use the same basic hardware setups. The pricing differences typically show up in the cost of the software, services and maintenance that the vendor provides to the practice. Some vendors will provide a discount on various components (e.g., discount licenses, lower the hourly service rate), while other vendors will offer a total system discount. Note that your comparison of price between two systems should include the maintenance fees over a certain evaluation period (e.g., 5 years). The key issue is the bottom price of the system (see **Chapter 7—Making a Final Decision**). To negotiate the price, you should have a detailed breakdown of the proposal, and insure that the "discount" is not based on cutting services or items that you will probably have to reinstate later. For example, one practice elected to have its training and implementation hours cut in half to "lower" the EMR cost. In another situation, a practice had to completely upgrade their hardware when they implemented the EMR under their combined PMS and EMR purchase.

Using the calculated delivered cost of the system (in **Chapter 7**), rework your estimate to account for the actual counts of users and the specifics of your situation. In some cases, you may need to contact the vendor to get specific details on the costs. For example, the software quote may contain several components for a fixed price or as a complete package. In some cases, vendors include a set number of hours in the software license cost. For example, a vendor may allow for up to 4 hours of training per license, but that may not be sufficient for a more complex organization.

Determine the differences between the final selection and the other products for which you calculated cost comparisons. Some EMR vendors have a single charge per user/provider while other vendors have a charge per module per user/provider. Unfortunately some EMR systems use a combination of charges. For example, they may charge per provider for the clinical content, per user for the EMR and per workstation for the scanning application. Verify the specific licenses you need to insure that you don't buy items you don't need. When in doubt, buy the lower quantity and include a clause in the contract that lets you buy additional licenses at the same price within a certain period of time. From a budgeting perspective, you should include the additional cost in a contingency fee.

In the pricing review, ensure that you consider the strategic plans and foreseeable events for your practice. For example, servicing another legal entity (e.g., therapy center, ASC) and adding providers could trigger unexpected charges that could substantially impact the price to the practice. After completing your working documents, consider the following issues:

- Is the package price hiding overpriced items?
- Are industry standard hardware and software items fairly priced?
- Does the hourly rate for various services favorably compare with other vendors?
- Were volume discounts received for a large numbers of licenses, service hours and workstations/tablets?
- Are maintenance and support charges discounted for the level of support directly provided by the practice?
- Was an additional discount available for purchasing or committing to purchase items that the practice may not need for a few months?

Warranties

A surprising number of EMR vendors provide little to no warranty. The typical contract states that the "Vendor provides NO WARRANTY." Vendors have a wide range of excuses for such terms, but your practice needs some assurance that the vendor will stand behind their product, solve you problems and allow you to rely on their EMR as the primary repository of patient information for your practice. Otherwise, you should find another EMR product.

Note that the promise to refund your money and de-install the system is not a practical resolution to a warranty issue. After you have started the implementation process, the cost of switching EMR products will dramatically increase for your practice. After the EMR is in use, switching to another EMR is almost impossible. The key to warranty issues remains the resolution of the problem to your satisfaction. The cost of backing out of the EMR for your practice may be too high for you to practically move to another product.

Warranties should cover a number of areas:

Software—The EMR Software should work with the hardware and within a functional standard. The functional standard should be easily referenced and reviewed. **ALERT:** Many EMR systems lack sufficient documentation to specify how the product works. Indeed, some areas of the product may be adequately documented and other features may lack any documentation.

Hardware—Hardware should work with the software and perform at a level that is needed by the practice. **ALERT:** If you are not buying the hardware from the EMR vendor, make sure that the hardware vendor is committed to the EMR requirements.

Services—Services should be provided by competent staff and the practice should be able to rely on their advice. Services should be provided at a level that is responsive to the practice. **TIP:** This warranty is important to insure that you do not have to pay for poor services and pay again to get the appropriate services.

Support—The support should be provided on a timely basis considering the problem, and support should be provided for a reasonable time after the practice has installed the EMR. **ALERT:** Many EMR vendors reserve the right to terminate support in a timeframe (Ex. 30 days) that would irreparably harm you practice and put your access to the EMR patient records at risk.

Support

Your support needs will vary with your internal capabilities and the abilities of your staff. In the course of negotiating business points, the practice should ensure that the correct level of support is accounted for and included in the contract. The level of support should include appropriate levels of training, phone, onsite and consultations on issues and problems.

Before you will be able to negotiate support, you should determine how you will support your EMR users. You may have an internal support person who filters all user issues and resolves most problems before ever going to the vendor. Some practices completely rely on the EMR vendor to support all users. Your support strategy can significantly affect your support costs.

Negotiating contract terms is a time consuming process. Justify your effort by ensuring the following business issues are pretty much complete before you deal with contract terms and conditions (Table 8.1):

TABLE 8.1

Business Point	Issue	Recommendation
License Costs	Vendors may license EMRs by server, practice, provider, location and/or user. Some vendors use complex combinations of these factors in the licensing and contract terms. For example, some vendors license by provider, but limit the number of users per provider. Other vendors require licenses for all workstations in your practice rather than licensing the users. A few vendors even require a separate licensing fee for each location. To measure the importance of the licensing costs, you need to develop a realistic projection of the number of providers and users. Once you determine the various doctors, clinical staff, billers, and administrative users that will access the EMR, make sure that the license costs support the user base. Note that some vendors differentiate between doctors, mid-level clinicians and non-clinical users. User classifications can have a substantial effect on the license costs. For example, PAs who support the doctors but do not bill for patient services under their own biller numbers may cost substantially less to license than PAs who bill for patient services. These license terms should be carefully evaluated in light of your strategic plans and options. For example, you may want to evaluate the impact of adding a location or a new modality to your practice.	Consider the size of your practice; negotiate a volume discount for the licenses. Negotiate a reduced license fee for part-time providers and mid-level staff. Negotiate terms to allow for an appropriate number of "fill-in" providers and staff. Negotiate price issues where the other products may have included an item that is a separate cost for the selected product. Accommodate your growth by allowing for future purchases at a preferred rate. Verify that the license will allow for the workstations, locations and users that will be needed to practically use the EMR in your practice.
Service Costs	EMR purchases include a variety of services: hardware installation, software installation, clinical content development, project management, training and consulting. Service costs may be quoted on an hourly or fixed cost basis. Your practice should have a clear understanding of the scope of the quoted services as well as the real level of services that will be needed to complete the EMR implementation. In some cases, vendor estimates are incorrect due to the lack of detailed knowledge of your practice or formulas that minimize hours to cut the purchase price. For example, practices without trained staff or effective EMR procedures may require more implementation and training services. Inject a dose of reality and develop an internal estimate that allows for adequate training and support for the practice and not just address an optimistic estimate. *TIP:* Make sure that you allow for sufficient internal support staff and time to fulfill your responsibilities for implementing the EMR. You should also review the level of services and allow for additional training and support services as the project proceeds. *TIP:* Monitor the level of available services and the estimate to complete to insure that you have allowed for sufficient vendor services.	Carefully review the scope of services to insure that the various tasks needed to support EMR implementation are included in the scope or accounted for by the practice. Lock in a favorable services rate for the duration of the EMR implementation. In the event that you need more services, the practice should not have to pay the standard (non-negotiated rate). Include a contingency cost in your internal EMR budget to allow for adequate services to complete the project.
Maintenance and Support Costs	Maintenance and support costs are typically based on a percentage of the hardware and software costs. Hardware maintenance includes troubleshooting problems and onsite maintenance of covered equipment. *ALERT:* Note that many warranties from hardware vendors do not allow for onsite services. Onsite services are typically available at an additional cost. Software maintenance includes updates (but not installation of updates or update training for staff), help desk support for selected members of your staff and technical support for problems.	Ensure that the hardware configuration minimizes risk of failures within your needs and expectations. Allow appropriate practice staff to contact the vendor for support. Include a response standard and competency standard for the vendor's help desk and support services.

Continued

Continued from previous page

Business Point	Issue	Recommendation
	In some cases, maintenance services include working with any member of your staff, while other vendors will only work with a limited number of key practice users. Many maintenance clauses include a variety of exclusions that may present problems. These exclusions could lead to problems or additional charges for maintenance services. For example, support outside of standard hours or support of third party software may not be included in the maintenance charges. Some support contracts exclude the interface with your PMS or diagnostic equipment. *ALERT:* In some cases, the EMR vendor will not support third party software even if the software was purchased with the EMR.	Negotiate a reduced rate based on the level of service that you are providing to your users. For example, if your practice has an internal help desk, you may be able to get a discount on the software maintenance services. Insure the EMR and/or hardware vendor stands behind the hardware.
Scope of Work	EMR implementation includes a wide range of efforts among many practice and outside resources (see **Chapter 9 – Implementing an EMR**). The practice should have a clear understanding of the specific work that is covered by the agreement and costs as well as the other necessary efforts by the practice or other vendors. Some vendors will provide a list of services that they will perform but fail to inform you of items that will be needed. In many cases, your responsibilities and vendor exclusions are buried in dense contract text. Before you buy into the scope of work with the vendor, ensure that you have identified the key tasks and who will be responsible for those tasks – otherwise you may get behind on your commitments and disrupt your EMR implementation. In some cases, client-based delays to the EMR implementation can lead to additional charges. *ALERT* – Many practices undertake EMR projects without selecting or identifying the practice resources that will be responsible for implementing the EMR. EMRs require active support and participation from the clinical and management staffs of the practice.	Use Chapter 9 to verify the services that are provided by the vendor. Note that you may choose to eliminate vendor services based on your other vendors and internal staff. Verify that the practice can meet the performance requirements in the contract for services. Itemize vendor service exclusions and identify practice resources and third party vendors that will be providing these resources. Allow for scheduled status meetings to monitor usage of services and progress.
Hardware Source	Your hardware purchase strategy should be accounted for in the business points. Since your vendor sells its software to many practices, it should be able to advise you on the hardware setup issues even if you are not buying the hardware from them. *TIP:* Some vendors have published hardware requirements for their systems. If your EMR vendor does not sell hardware, it should specify the hardware requirements for all components in your system. In some cases, the vendor specifies specific models. In any event, verify any hardware purchases with the software vendor. If your EMR vendor sells hardware, you should seriously consider buying at least the EMR server with the software. Thereby, the EMR vendor is fully responsible for the main system that contains the EMR and you are free to buy the other hardware from another party.	Include the hardware and communication requirements from the software vendor in the contract. Software vendor should warrant that the recommended hardware will handle the practice workload. At a minimum, buy the EMR server from the EMR vendor. If the software vendor is selling the hardware to the practice, the hardware and software purchase should be connected in the warranty, payment plan and implementation plan.
Electronic Clearing-houses	Electronic transactions and clearinghouses are an evolving issue for EMRs. Several HIPAA Transactions (Claim Information, Electronic Prescriptions, and Referral/ PreCertification/ PreAuthorization) and the Continuity of Care Transaction require an electronic link to a clearinghouse for the EMR.	Ensure that the vendor is committed to supporting the transactions as needed by the practice.

Continued

Continued from previous page

Business Point	Issue	Recommendation
	Although clearinghouse use is an evolving issue for EMRs, you should be informed of the requirements for such exchanges and what support may be needed for exchanges with your key business partners.	Verify that the vendor's clearinghouse or direct connections support exchanges with your key healthcare partners (payers, pharmacies, hospitals). Verify that electronic prescriptions feature and clearinghouse works with the local pharmacies.
Timeline	EMR Vendors frequently want to defer any discussion on timelines until the contract is completed. Vendors do not want to commit their resources to a project that may not happen. However, you may have a pressing need to install the system by a certain time due to an office move, seasonal volume or some other obligation. On the other hand, the vendor may plan to implement the system in a timeframe that does not consider your needs and situation. If you have a tight schedule and have yet to complete the contract, consider negotiating a commitment letter with the vendor to get on the vendor's schedule.	Include key goal dates in the contract to insure the vendor will meet your scheduling needs and issues. Include a procedure for changing the goal dates at the practice's option. Compile an internal implementation plan to determine such dates and ensure that you have the resources to meet the goal dates.
Clinical Content	Clinical content consists of the templates, documents, knowledge-base and/or forms that you will use with the EMR. In some cases, vendors provide a very specific set of clinical content. Other vendors include all of the clinical content in their product. Some vendors provide access to a library of clinical content developed by other practices or sell clinical content from other vendors. You should make sure that the purchase agreement includes the various clinical content areas that you need for your practice and expect in the EMR. You should be especially careful to include clinical content that you may have considered in your review of EMR products. For example, you may have seen clinical templates during a site visit or in the vendor's web site that was a significant contributor to the product decision. In some cases, the vendor will be developing the clinical content. For example, an EMR product may lack clinical content in your specialty and the vendor has offered to develop the clinical content with the understanding that it will add the content to its product. In the event that your practice is developing clinical content, you should have a clear understanding of the ownership of the clinical content and maintenance responsibilities. In some cases, vendors reserve the right to offer your clinical content to other practices. If you have a problem allowing other practices to use your templates, then the business arrangement should prevent the distribution of your templates.	Insure that the clinical content to be delivered with the product is included in the contract. For example, a primary care practice with cardiology specialists will need the cardiology content *and* the primary care content. *TIP:* For vendors that charge for clinical content, make sure that you arrange for your foreseeable needs. You are in a stronger negotiating and discount position when you are originally buying the EMR than when you try to add additional items later. If you will be developing clinical content, specify what assistance the vendor will provide as well as the disposition of the final clinical content. If the vendor is developing clinical content for your practice to enhance its own product, ensure that you have defined the scope of the clinical content, a timeline to meet your needs and a support commitment from the vendor. Itemize the clinical content that will be included in the purchase and/or sources of necessary clinical content.
Training Strategy	Depending on the size of your organization, you may have the vendor train selected staff and then have the selected staff train the rest of the practice or you may have the vendor train all of your staff. The training class location is also part of the training strategy.	Include the training plan and strategy in the contract.

Continued

Continued from previous page

Business Point	Issue	Recommendation
	Training typically is split up into (1) setup training and (2) application training. Setup training addresses how you establish the various lists, shortcuts, templates and documents using the administrative and programming capabilities of the EMR. Application training focuses on the actual use of the EMR to track patients, chart visits and manage work. In some cases, vendors offer advanced training to teach additional features as well as programming of the clinical content. Vendors vary in their training strategies. Some vendors insist that you attend EMR training at their training centers. Others are just as committed to conducting training at your location. The training location should be determined during the contract negotiations to ensure that you contract for the services you need and that the contract accounts for the costs at the selected location. Training at vendor offices is typically based on a per day/student charge, while onsite training is based on a charge per day/per trainer. Several vendors offer web-based training and access to web training broadcasts. A combination of these training options will be used to complete the EMR effort.	Select the venue for training. Allow for access to web-based training facilities for all staff and doctors. Identify the specific materials that will be provided to the practice in support of the training and implementation process.

When you have agreed to the business points with the vendor, then you are ready to work on the specific contract terms that will reflect the business agreement that you have reached as well as ensure a results-oriented working arrangement with the EMR vendor. Check business issues against the contract terms as you conduct contract negotiations. Be careful to preserve the business deal and not include specific terms that undermine or change the basic arrangement with the software vendor. For example, you may negotiate a training plan that is directly contradicted by the standard contract terms.

NEGOTIATING CONTRACT TERMS

EMR contracts widely range in complexity and terms. Each vendor has a different focus and issues that will be conveyed in its contract language. Some vendors may provide you with several agreements. For example, you may have a software license, support agreement and hardware agreement to evaluate and sign to buy the vendor's product as well as a license from the owner of the EMR software. You need to carefully review each agreement to insure it consistently and appropriately meets your needs.

Guide your contracting efforts by the following principles:

The vendor contract was written for the vendor—Vendor contracts are written by the vendor's lawyers to protect the vendor from losses, and limit its exposure. In general, vendors have a legitimate concern that someone will steal their ideas and strategies, but the terms that they impose can cause serious operational problems or easily place the practice in technical violation of the contract. As you will see in Table 8.2, vendor contracts contain a wide range of terms and conditions that can make your life difficult and expose you to unnecessary risks.

Everything is negotiable—EMR software vendors want your business. The sales people will typically not want to walk away from a potential customer because you will not agree to little protection for you investment. The vast majority of EMR vendors will work with you to develop a workable agreement.

You are not the only person to have a problem with the contract—Some vendors will tell you that everyone signs his contracts as is, and that they fail to understand what the problem is. However, you are often dealing with a company that is not local, and your practice could pay the price for a delay or disruption in the implementation or use of an EMR. Whether anyone else has a problem or not is not the issue: you are the one who will have to work within the terms of the contract.

Remember that you will have to live with the contract structure for as long as you use its EMR. As such, you need to establish a results-oriented relationship that will provide you with the structure to establish and manage a continuing relationship with the vendor. The following table itemizes the key contract issues and presents a mitigation strategy for these key issues. Note that EMR contracts may contain a number of other issues that you will have to address, too (see Table 8.2).

WORKING ON THE FINAL AGREEMENT

As you negotiate the contract with the vendor, you will go through several iterations of text. Some vendors will add the changes into the body of the contract, while others will create an addendum that will be attached to the basic contract. Changes in words, concepts and terms throughout the contracting process could affect other areas. To manage the contracting process, compile a list of issues.

To keep things simple, make sure that all changes are tracked and be on guard for unexpected additions and changes. For example, one vendor added contract items that contradicted other contract terms. Another vendor unilaterally made changes to a final copy of the contract to "clean up the language." In both cases, the changes would have substantially changed the nature of the contract and the agreement. Successfully manage the negotiations by considering the following:

Maintain an Issues List—When the contract is initially reviewed, compile a list of issues and your desired outcome. The issues list should be used to track your progress and outstanding items. Make sure you identify which items are negotiable versus items that you view as less important. You do not want to spend a lot of time and effort addressing a minor issue and then have to compromise on a more important item. Note that you should include your business points in the issues list. Frequently, a contract change will undermine or change a business point that has already been addressed. For example, the vendor may introduce a new term to deal with your problem, but creates ambiguous language in other sections of the contract. When your contract issue is to align the contract with the business point, vendors are typically more accommodating.

TABLE 8.2

Contract Issues	Issue	Typical Contract Text	Mitigation Strategy
Access to the System	Many EMR contracts severely limit the types of people who can access your system. Contracts may limit access to your employees, employees who "need access," or some other measure. In some cases, the vendor demands that it be informed of who has access to the system and/or require people with access to sign an agreement with the vendor. Such a term is a severe impediment to your practice. Your practice may need to make the system available to consultants, contract physicians or prospective physicians and employees. You need to be able to pursue your practice's objectives without worrying about approvals from you EMR vendors or risking violating your contract. Note that many contacts with system access limitations will terminate your software licenses for failure to follow the procedures in its contracts.	Practice will provide system access solely to your employees Practice will provide system access to employees who have agreed to the conditions of this contract. Any party with access to the system will have signed the attached agreement.	Allow the practice to disclose information about the EMR system and provide access to the EMR system to pursue the business or service objectives of the practice. Permit the practice to provide screen shots and reports as needed to pursue patient service and business needs of the practice.
Additional Charges	Vendor contracts frequently specify a wide range of situations where additional charges may be incurred. Travel expenses are typically classified as additional charges. Off-hours support, questions from unauthorized staff (in the vendor's eyes, but necessary staff for your practice), excessive support according to the vendor, and information available from manuals may trigger additional charges. Some vendors even reserve the right to charge for support issues after they fix the problem. The practice needs to insure that additional charges are cost effective and authorized. For example, you may not want off-hours support for a non-critical issue that can be addressed during regular hours.	Vendor may charge for support services that it determines, in vendor's sole discretion, to be excessive. Support is limited to 2 hours of phone support per month. Additional time will be charged to the practice. Other charges will be billed when incurred. Bills for other charges are due upon receipt. Services must be provided by the Go Live date.	Include an estimate of additional charges that are expected for the project. Travel, communications, wiring expenses and other expenses not included in the contract should be estimated by the vendor. Require additional charges to be approved in writing by the practice. Manage the project to include periodic reviews of the remaining hours and an estimate of hours needed to complete the project. Insure that the contract allows you to switch unused hours from one category to another category as the project proceeds. Insure that additional charges are controlled and capped.
Assignment of License	Medical practices may merge or reorganize under another practice structure. Since the practice has already paid for the license, the inability to assign the license could lead to additional charges or a new license fee.	Non-assignable License License may not be assigned to any party.	Allow assignment of the license as part of a merger or reorganization of the practice without any additional charges. Assignment of the license should only require notification to and not approval of the vendor. Assignment of the license should allow for assignment of all rights for the software, support and other rights.

Continued

Continued from previous page

Contract Issues	Issue	Typical Contract Text	Mitigation Strategy
	Vendors claim that the clause prevents competitors from buying their product, but the practical effect is to expose the practice to additional charges or the loss of the license to use the EMR. For example, an unassignable license could not be assigned to an organization that acquires your practice or a spin off of your billing operation.		
Bill Payment	Most vendor contracts compel you to pay bills under the threat of losing your license or having support services withdrawn. Although you should pay justifiable bills, the lack of warranties in most contracts limits your power to compel the vendor to perform or seek redress for incorrect billing, and/or billing adjustments. In the absence of a dispute mechanism, your practice is at risk whenever you may dispute a charge. Unfortunately, problems with bills are fairly frequent and include early-support billing, billing for undelivered items and billing for unsatisfactory and unauthorized services. In many cases, vendors are difficult to work with on billing issues. They are impossible when the contract does not allow for billing disputes.	Failure to pay any bills is considered breach of the license. All bills are due upon receipt.	Establish a bill-dispute procedure to allow the practice to reasonably dispute bills without risking any problems or penalties. Establish a performance standard that allows the practice to dispute a bill in the event of unsatisfactory services. Allow for verification and acceptance of products and services in the contract. For example, you may pay the bill for the interface after you have tested the EMR interface with the PMS.
Business Associate Agreement	The Business Associate Agreement is a HIPAA Privacy issue that controls what the vendor needs to do to protect your health information in the EMR. **Beware:** Many vendors do not present the Business Associate Agreement until after the contract has been signed. Fortunately, many Business Associate Agreements are fairly compliant with the HIPAA Privacy requirements. Nonetheless, you should insure that the BA is acceptable and that the agreement is signed with the contract.	In many cases, the contract does not reference the Business Associate Agreement.	Contemporaneously review, negotiate and sign the Business Associate Agreement with the EMR purchase contract.
Clinical Content	Many EMR systems offer clinical content, templates and documents for your area of practice and specialty (See Business Points Above.) However, some vendors are presenting clinical content that is not included, sold by another entity or not operational.	EMR is sold as is. No mention of clinical content in the contract. Practice can use (unspecified) clinical content available on the vendor website.	Insure that the specified clinical content is included in the contract. For example, the contract may specify a content package or clinical area that will be included in the purchase.

Continued

Continued from previous page

Contract Issues	Issue	Typical Contract Text	Mitigation Strategy
	Many contracts address the ownership and support for the clinical content. Options range from vendors that provide a complete panel of clinical content to vendors that provide a toolkit that allows you to develop your own clinical content using their toolkit. Some vendors provide only access to clinical content that have been developed by other practices. The clinical content from other practices can be downloaded to your system and installed in your EMR. If the EMR vendor develops content for you, the vendor frequently reserves the right to provide or sell the templates to other practices.	Templates and documents developed by the vendor or practice can be sold or provided to other practices without compensation to the practice.	If the clinical content is a key requirement, you may want to itemize the clinical content that is included in the purchase as well as a delivery and installation mechanism for your purchase. Allow for access and use of additional clinical content based on additional services provided by the practice. Include updates to clinical content as part of the support agreement. If desired, limit use of templates, documents and other clinical content developed by or for your practice as confidential information. Limits on distribution may be especially important for practices that develop specific clinical content to support a proprietary process that is important to your practice.
Communication Requirements	EMRs will generate more data exchanges with remote offices than anything you have done to date. EMRs collect more information for a visit that a PMS and the use of images will push the level of communications far beyond your current connection. The vendor should indicate the bandwidth level needed to support the number of workstations and necessary connections at each location. The Practice should be especially careful with the communication requirements needed to support scanning of documents on a day-to-day basis as well as the volume of scanning for legacy paper charts. *TIP:* Due to the lead time for communication upgrades, your should make sure that your order the communication services in time to meet your EMR implementation plan.	Practice is responsible for adequate communications between remote sites and the server. Practice must provide adequate communication access to the EMR server for the vendor.	Include specifications for necessary communications between the practice locations. Specify what, if any, communications will be necessary for vendor access. Insure that the delivery of communications will be in time to support other vendor activities, such as testing and training. Review the image scanning and management requirements for the EMR. For example, some EMRs burst the images, which may require a higher bandwidth.
Confidential Information	Confidential information consists of the policies, procedures, processes, forms and practices of your practice. In many EMR contracts, you are obligated to protect the EMR vendor's confidential information, but most vendors do not have a reciprocal obligation to protect your confidential information. A vendor could take materials from your practice and provide those materials to other vendor customers. If you have a specific workflow process or clinical content that you consider proprietary, you will want to limit the distribution of these materials.	All vendor information including documentation, flowcharts, screen shots and documents are considered confidential information. Practice may not provide confidential information to any party except authorized practice employees.	Limit vendor use of any and all information related to practices' procedures, business practices, clinical strategies, contractual relationships and any patient information. Prevent distribution of any practice information that could help a competitor. For example, promotional strategies and marketing channels, as well as suppliers may be proprietary information.

Continued

Continued from previous page

Contract Issues	Issue	Typical Contract Text	Mitigation Strategy
	Depending on the importance of the policies, procedures and other confidential information, you may want to restrict their use by the vendor.		
Customization	Some EMRs include customization services. Customization services may include adding clinical content or the development of an entire set of screens to support a specialty that the vendor currently lacks. If a lot of customization is required, you should consider an initial project to specify the changes before you buy the product. The vendor can show you mock-ups or initial screens of the EMR before you buy. And the vendor will be able to specify the costs of the effort as well as the delivery time. EMR customization should be subject to an acceptance and testing process. The process may include testing of actual patient information as well as a warranty period to cover the initial EMR use. **ALERT:** In some cases, you may implement adjustments to the vendor's clinical content to meet your needs. Those changes may have to be reinstalled to future vendor releases, or you may have to forgo use of the vendor's standard clinical content.	Vendor will develop clinical templates for the practice on a time and materials basis. Vendor provides NO WARRANTY.	Specify the scope of the customization effort. Scope documents may include lists of functions, screen mockups and descriptions. A standard of performance or functionality should be included in the Agreement. Include a cost estimate or fixed price. Define a testing and acceptance process for the customization effort. The testing process should include documenting patient visits from existing patient charts, as well as live shadowing of patient encounters. Include support for customized components (e.g., interfaces, and clinical content) in vendor support responsibilities.
Documentation	Most EMR contracts limit the use of the documentation in the same manner that the access to the system is controlled. You may not be able to copy the documentation or present the documentation to people who are not authorized users. You may want to make extensive use of the documentation. You may need to provide documentation on the system to outside clinical chart review consultants and quality assurance staff from a key payer. You may need to use the documentation to develop the procedures and processes that are required under the HIPAA Privacy and Security standards.	Cannot copy documentation for any reason. Documentation cannot be provided to anyone who is not an employee of the practice.	Allow the practice to copy, store, duplicate, and use the documentation to pursue the business purpose of the practice. Permit use of copies of documentation in procedure manuals and other practice operational materials. After the practice stops using the system, the documentation should be retained by the practice to assure continuity of medical record information and access to the purchased EMR.

Continued

Continued from previous page

Contract Issues	Issue	Typical Contract Text	Mitigation Strategy
Electronic Data Interchange	Electronic data interchange (EDI) involves the exchange of electronic data between various healthcare organizations. Currently, EMRs may send electronic prescriptions to selected pharmacies. In the future, EDI will support the exchange of information on patient treatment, clinical records and the Continuity of Care Record (CCR.) The key issue is the ability of the system to support the sending and receiving of transactions and the mode of transmission (e.g., clearinghouse, direct). Although many EMR systems do not support these capabilities currently, the practice should have a clear understanding of its options.	Vendor supports EDI with the ABC Clearinghouse. All electronic transactions are router to the vendor's clearinghouse.	Insure that the vendor supports current transactions including electronic prescriptions. Include a clause that commits to the support of industry standard transactions such as the Continuity of Care Record, and the Additional Claim Information HIPAA Transaction. Commit vendor to supporting exchanges with key payers, hospitals and providers. Note that some vendors will specify the HL-7 transaction format for the electronic exchange of information with other parties. Such a standard is a reasonable approach for electronic exchanges.
EMR Support	Typically, EMR support consists of problem-solving resources as well as the right to receive future updates. However, some vendors charge additional fees for future updates. For example, the vendor may reserve the right to add a surcharge for future updates, or split the product into modules which must be purchased by the practice to continue to have access to current functionality. Some EMR vendors require that you upgrade to the newest version of their product within a certain calendar period or until a specific number of new versions have been released. Support terms frequently control who can contact the vendor, what the vendor will do and the obligations of the practice. For example, some vendors exclude support for third-party products that may be an integral part of your EMR. For example, the EMR may use a third-party drawing tool that is built into the EMR. If the vendor runs into a problem with the third-party software, you may have to cope with reduced functionality or performance problems. Other vendors may only authorize a specific employee to contact the vendor support staff.	Support services consist of phone support to designated users and distributions of updates to the EMR that the vendor may release from time to time at its sole discretion. EMR support fees may be increased with 60-days notice. Phone support provided to designated users. EMR updates may be released at vendor's discretion. Practice will update its EMR to the current version of the software within 30 days of software version release. Vendor will only support the current release of the EMR software.	Insure continuous vendor support of the EMR product for at least 5 years after the practice installs the EMR. Vendors should not be able to terminate support for any reason during that period. Notice of support termination should be provided by the EMR vendor at least 18 months before support ceases. This gives your practice time to move to another EMR product. Limit support fee increases to a specific percentage or standard (e.g., CPI or consumer price index). Establish a support performance standard. The standard should include a response requirement for critical problems and system failures. Installation of the current version of the product can be delayed by the practice for a reasonable period of time. Support for the previous version or two previous versions of the EMR software will be provided by the vendor for a period of time that would allow the practice to review and test the new EMR software version.

Continued

Continued from previous page

Contract Issues	Issue	Typical Contract Text	Mitigation Strategy
	In some cases, EMR support is a requirement for continuing use of the EMR. If you terminate support, the vendor terminates your license. As a practical matter, you may terminate EMR support when you stop using the EMR but the practice may still need to access old EMR records for years after the switch. If you have to continue support to get access to the EMR and patient records after you stop using the software, your practice may have to pay thousands of dollars a year for an indefinite period of time.		
Entity	The contracting entity may be a significant issue for the contract. If you are a single corporation, LLC or other entity, the contracting entity is the practice. If you have several entities, including a clinical practice and other entities (e.g., ASC, optical shop, physical therapy), then you need to insure that the various entities are included in the contract.	EMR may only be used to serve the customer. Exclusive agreement between the customer and vendor.	Include all relevant practice entities in the contract term. Add a term to allow the practice to use the EMR with its related entities. List the related entities that will use the EMR in the contract.
Environment	Many vendors stipulate general requirements for the computer location and support. Vendors may include power, air conditioning and access requirements. Note that the environmental issues may be impacted by your hardware vendor source. For example, the EMR server may be installed in a rack provided by your normal hardware vendor. To insure continuity of operations and reliable access to your EMR, you should follow the appropriate vendor guidelines but add in an additional standard to mitigate the risk of an EMR failure (**see Chapter 9 – Implementing an EMR**).	Practice must maintain the computer equipment in an appropriate space with adequate utilities and ventilation. Vendor must be able to access the system at any time without impediment.	Include the vendor's standards in the contract. Then you may have recourse for a performance or sizing problem. Insure that the vendor agrees to your equipment and hardware setup. Verify that you are in compliance with the vendor's specified standards. Analyze the vendor standards in light of the HIPAA Security standards. If necessary, negotiate down issues that exceed the HIPAA Security Requirements.
Error Definition	Most vendor contracts address errors that your practice may encounter. Unfortunately, many contracts provide wide latitude to the vendor in acknowledging an error. Some contracts require a reporting window, while others exclude problems as a result of data "entered" by the practice. It is difficult to image that an error would not be triggered by practice data.	Vendor will fix errors that the vendor determines is not consistent with the operation of the system. Vendor will not fix problems that are caused by practice data.	Include a clause that establishes a reference standard for the operation of the software. Potential standards could include the manual or what a user could "reasonably expect" from the system. If the performance standard is online documentation, make sure that you print the supporting documentation in support of any errors. In some cases, conflicting documentation has disappeared or the vendor has "fixed the documentation."

Continued

Continued from previous page

Contract Issues	Issue	Typical Contract Text	Mitigation Strategy
	The best strategy is to include a defined standard against which errors will be measured. The standard may include documentation, industry practices or a "reasonable" expectation.	Vendor may fix the error or amend the documentation.	Note that some EMR product documentation generally lacks the specific performance or description that would support your practice in a dispute. Make sure that you fully understand the quality of the documentation and how it may be used to support any functionality and performance issues. Error correction should be performed on a best-effort basis for errors that effect the day-to-day operations of the practice. Require written-practice approval for error correction charges by the vendor. Such a process should allow for a testing phase before using the corrected software in your live database.
Exit Strategy.	Vendor contracts are written to describe the early stages of your project and the implementation effort. In the event of a license problem, contract dispute, product obsolescence or your decision to move to a new EMR in the future, your practice needs to allow for a smooth transition to another EMR. Your practice will also need continued access to the existing EMR for reference purposes. If you were to move to another EMR, you will have to deal with a project that is many times more complex and demanding than any PMS conversion. To understand the magnitude of the problem, you should note that many PMS vendors will not accommodate conversion of patient ledger details. Will your practice be able to function without your prescription list, or procedure list from the "old" EMR? Imagine the difficulty you would have if you could not access or had EMR information split among two EMR systems. Such a situation may prevent you from maintaining the "Designated Record Set" mandated by the HIPAA Privacy Standards.	Practice may terminate the use of the software with X days notice. The practice will discontinue use of the software and destroy all copies of the software.	Insure that the vendor will support the conversion of practice EMR data, when and if the practice moves to another EMR. Regardless of the reason for moving to another EMR, allow continuous practice access to the EMR system and data for as long as the practice needs. Such access may be needed to check the original medical record data that was brought over from the old EMR. The ability to access the old EMR should be available for as long as the practice deems necessary. Access to the old data should not be contingent on paying continuing support costs.
Hardware Support	A hardware failure could be a localized issue or a complete shutdown of your facility. The best strategy for hardware support is to invest in hardware that minimizes potential failure.	Hardware support will be provided by vendor through a third party organization of the vendor's choosing.	Support will be provided by the EMR vendor to assist in the analysis of hardware issues on a best effort basis.

Continued

Contract Issues	Issue	Typical Contract Text	Mitigation Strategy
	Cost effective options should be considered in light of your risk of loss and operational issues (see **Chapter 7 – Making a Final Decision**). Some practices have no tolerance for an EMR loss and other practices can tolerate a brief loss of the EMR system. A number of cost effective hardware investments include a high availability cluster server(s) with redundant disk arrays, power supplies, fans and other components. Additional system redundancies can be purchased to control the risk of a complete system failure. Nonetheless, you should insure that the hardware support accommodates a level of risk that you can live with. For example, if you purchase a system with several redundant components, an 8-hour response may be acceptable. But another practice may seek a 2-hour response and/or invest in more system redundancy.	Onsite hardware support will be provided within one business day of the support call. Hardware calls should be placed to the practice hardware vendor. The EMR vendor support line will address only software issues.	Provide onsite hardware support services within 4 hours of a hardware support call or some other response rate that meets the practice's needs. Allow for additional EMR vendor hardware support outside of standard business hours as needed. Specify onsite hardware sparing requirements to shorten recovery time.
HIPAA Compliance	If your Practice is a covered entity, then you need to comply with the HIPAA Privacy, Security and Transaction standards. Many vendor contracts are silent on the support of HIPAA standards. Practices will be under increasing pressure to support electronic interfaces with other healthcare organizations. Many of these exchanges will be based on the HIPAA Transaction Set. HIPAA Transactions include several exchanges that will require an EMR. The practice should insure that the vendor will support appropriate HIPAA transactions. The HIPAA Privacy standard specifies tracking disclosures and the paperwork needed to support such disclosures. Since many disclosure of Protected Health Information will come from the EMR, the EMR should support tracking and managing disclosures.	Software product will be maintained to meet applicable state and federal laws.	Maintain the Software product to meet the current HIPAA Privacy, Security and Transaction Requirements. Insure that vendor warrants that the software will enable the practice to comply with the HIPAA Privacy Standards, HIPAA Security Standards and use the relevant HIPAA Transaction Sets. Insure that Vendor will supply appropriate communication and transaction processing facilities to allow practice to use the EMR to formulate and process appropriate HIPAA Transactions.
Interfaces – Diagnostic	Interfaces support the exchange of information with other software products or systems. An EMR may need to interface with the PMS, lab system, reference labs, diagnostic equipment and other provider systems. For example, the practice may have an EKG machine that produces electronic images.	Many contracts are silent on these interfaces. Interfaces may be included in the purchase order.	Compile a list of the diagnostic equipment in your practice. Verify the electronic interface between the diagnostic equipment and the EMR. Identify the strategy and components needed to get the diagnostic information into the EMR.

Continued

Continued from previous page

Contract Issues	Issue	Typical Contract Text	Mitigation Strategy
	Some diagnostic equipment supports direct interfaces with other systems. For example, the diagnostic equipment may produce an image that can be accepted into the EMR.		Include diagnostic equipment interface products, and, if necessary, custom interfaces in the purchase order. Include services needed from the vendor to get the interfaces to work with your equipment.
Interfaces – Lab	EMRs accept lab orders during the patient visit. Depending on the capabilities of the EMR, the lab orders may be electronically transmitted to selected reference labs, and the results returned electronically to the EMR. Note that some reference labs subsidize the purchase of the lab interface.	EMR includes an interface with reference labs specified in the purchase order.	Verify that the lab interface works with the local office of your key reference labs. Insure that the purchase order allows for the lab interface module as well as the services to test, use and support the lab interface.
Interfaces – PMS	If you are buying an integrated system, you have no interface issues. If you have an existing PMS that you will be integrating with your EMR, the contract should include a commitment to support and maintain the interface with the PMS. *ALERT:* Even if you are buying the EMR from your PMS vendor, you may need to insure that the product interface will continue to be maintained. If you are interfacing your EMR with your PMS, you want to insure that you have such an option in the future. If you plan to replace your PMS at a future date, the EMR contract should accommodate the purchase and implementation of the future interface.	EMR does not include interfaces with any products. Interfaces are the responsibility of the practice	Itemize the interfaces supported by the PMS interface (e.g., demographics, appointments, charges) with the EMR. Include the interface software as well as a warranty and support arrangement for the interface. If the PMS interface is not a standard product, include a warranty and defined standard for the operation and speed of the interface. For example, the EMR should post demographic and appointment information from the PMS within 5 seconds of receipt of an interface transaction. If no PMS interface is being implemented, include a term that allows for such an interface in the future. The item may even include selected products or interface standards (e.g., HL7).
Key Contacts	Before the contract is signed, you will be working with the sales team. After the contract is signed, most vendors turn the practice over to the implementation team. In many cases, you have not met the implementation staff. If possible, try to meet the implementation manager and key trainer *before* signing the contract. Otherwise, reserve the right to approve the key staff and insure that adequate warranties are in place to assure competency.	Vendor will staff the contract with qualified employees and/or third party resources.	Identify the vendor project manager and other key people for the EMR implementation. Reserve the right to approve the project manager after an initial interview. In the event of a change in key vendor personnel on the project, reserve the right to interview replacement vendor staff. If the change was driven by the vendor, the practice should not have to pay additional money to get the new staff member up to speed on the project.

Continued

Continued from previous page

Contract Issues	Issue	Typical Contract Text	Mitigation Strategy
Licenses	Vendors may offer a license to use the EMR for a set period of time (say, 5 years) or subject its use to other conditions, including locations and placement of the server. As a practical matter, the practice should be certain that the license does not include limitations that are not practical, or may be overlooked as the practice pursues its objectives. Be especially careful to avoid license terms that require additional payment and unexpected approvals from the EMR Vendor.	Practice is buying a non-exclusive license to use the software for X years. Practice may use the software for as long as the practice pays monthly support fees.	Insure that licenses for a set period clearly state the renewal terms and conditions. In the event of license termination or non-renewal, the vendor must support the exit strategy.
Patents and Copyrights	Vendor contracts include terms to protect their intellectual property rights over the design, interface and other EMR aspects. Most vendor contracts include terms that protect the vendor in the event of a competing copyright or patent claim. Typically, the vendor will try to reach a licensing agreement, change the EMR product or remove the offending software/feature. Removal of the software/feature is an unacceptable outcome since your practice may depend on the eliminated item. Even a refund of a portion of the license fees is unacceptable. The vendor should address the legal issue without affecting your practice's EMR capability.	In the event of a ruling against the vendor, the vendor may pay a license fee to the patent holder, change the feature to remove the infringement or remove the feature from the software.	Insure vendor uses its best efforts to make sure the practice has continued access to the feature or EMR. Prevent vendor from avoiding the problem by paying a portion of the license fees back to the practice. Verify changes to comply with copyright claims do not increase the complexity of using the product or the feature.
Payment Schedule	Vendors typically seek to get a substantial payment upfront and the rest of the money before you have a chance to see the EMR. Indeed, some contracts have you paying remaining charges upon the delivery of boxes containing your EMR components. Unfortunately, you cannot go too far with a box of components. Ideally, the vendor should be paid based on performance and your receipt of value. Key payment triggers to consider are when the hardware and software are available for use, completion of training, and Go Live of the EMR. If the purchase includes customization services, then some payment may be appropriate after you have tested and accepted the changes.	Practice will pay 50% of the total contract at the signing of the contract and the remaining 50% when the products are shipped from the vendor's office.	Minimize the payment at contract signing. Pay a portion of the fee at delivery defined as the software is available for use and working with your workstations and tablets. This term may require coordination with your hardware vendor. Pay for time and expense charges as the charges are incurred. Allow for fixed price or volume buy services to be used beyond the Go Live date.

Continued

Continued from previous page

Contract Issues	Issue	Typical Contract Text	Mitigation Strategy
Performance Standards	A wide variety of variables can impact the performance of the system and the software. The capacity of the communication lines, your hardware base, network setup and other user activities can effect how quickly the system responds to a user. Nonetheless, you should seek to establish a base performance level to set your expectation as well as to commit the vendor to work with you on any performance issues. Performance issues will be based on the hardware and software setup recommendations of the Vendor, as well as what other users are doing with the system.	Vendor makes NO WARRANTIES.	The recommended hardware and software should produce a response time to a workstation request of no more than X seconds.
Providers	Many vendors base license charges on a provider. However, many practices employ various "providers" – such as nurse practitioners and physician assistants – who exclusively assist the doctor and part-time providers. Paying a full license amount for all providers could result in substantial fee to the practice. The definition of a provider is an important factor to consider. The practice should seriously review the current list of providers as well as future plans to insure that you do not pay for provider licenses for those providers who work less than full time or under supervision.	A provider is anyone involved in clinical decision making for patients. A provider is a doctor, nurse, LPN or other licensed healthcare professional.	Define a provider considering your clinical staff. The contract should itemize special situations including supporting PA/LPN/RN, technicians and other clinicians who provide limited independent patient services. Allow for licenses to be shared by providers who are not full-time providers or may fill in for the doctors. For example, the practice may employ fill-in providers on an as-needed basis. The practice should be able to give access to fill-in providers without paying a full license fee for each provider. Allow for a reporting and authorization process that is not difficult and can respond to the practice's need to provide quick access to fill-in doctors/staff.
Services Purchased	An EMR contract may include a variety of services based on different charge methods. Services may be based on a time-and-expenses basis or a fixed-price basis. Service charges may vary by method (e.g., onsite, offsite, phone, Internet). Note that many service proposals look like fixed- price proposals, when they're really time and materials agreements. You should verify that the contract services are sufficient and appropriate for the practice.	Full payment will be made when the system is delivered. Services will be provided by vendor staff or third parties as needed. Services include training, implementation, project management and other efforts in support of the practice.	Services should be paid as incurred. Carefully review the scope of work to manage the use of hours and fixed price exclusions. Include an option to purchase additional services at a negotiated project rate. Insure that the mix of services is reasonable for the practice. Include a periodic review process to track the services provided by the vendor and the progress of the project. Allow for swapping services among the various areas as needed during the project. For example, leftover training hours could be used to purchase more practice management services.

Continued

Continued from previous page

Contract Issues	Issue	Typical Contract Text	Mitigation Strategy
Software Requirements	In some cases, practices have some critical EMR functionality that is an absolute necessity for success. In the course of demonstrations, the Practice may have the impression that the EMR product meets the requirement. Unfortunately, some practices find out that they didn't buy what they saw or the product demonstration showed an impractical workaround. If the product has the critical item currently, you may want to highlight the requirement in the contract. If the product lacks the function and the vendor has promised to add the capability, or do some custom work, then the strategy and function should be specified in the contract with a completion or delivery date.	Product is sold as is without any representation that the software will meet the practice's needs. Practice understands the specific capabilities of the EMR Product. Practice is solely responsible for determining that the EMR product meets the practice's needs.	Itemize the critical functionality and/or feature as a primary reason for the purchase of the EMR. The itemization should include a description of the capability sufficient to understand the requirement and process. Verify that the product handles the issue to the practice's satisfaction or itemize the changes and delivery schedule for the enhancement.
Source Code Escrow	The EMR program is based on source code that is owned by the software publisher. The source code normally is not stored on your system. However, source code is needed to make changes and fix bugs. Some vendors have an established escrow agreement that gives you access to the source code in the event of bankruptcy or business failure. Note that access to source may not be as comforting as you think, since the source code would have to be studied by trained programmers before they could help you make changes or fix problems.	Source code is the property of the vendor. Source code is not included in the purchase of the software.	Insure that the vendor supports an escrow program with an established agent (setting your own escrow facility up is a more expensive and complex task). Determine the frequency and currency of the escrow program in light of the EMR product releases. Participate in the vendor's escrow program.
System Activation	System activation or "Go Live" drives a variety of issues and services. Vendors may turn the support over to the vendor's support team, require the start of support payments and/or stop project management services. In the case of EMRs, you may spend several months setting up the system to be used while the vendor may consider the system activated when the system is delivered in boxes or when the EMR server has been connected to your computer network. In other cases, you may actually be using the system to scan old charts and track patient messages, but be months away from the charting of patient visits by doctor. You need to make sure that you have continuing support to carry you through to actual use of the EMR.	System will be considered activated or Go Live when the purchased items are delivered. Practice will pay in full when the EMR is available for use.	Activation should be defined as the point in time when your practice is using the system for productive work. For example, activation could be defined when the staff has been trained and doctors are using the system to chart patient services. Activation can trigger payments as well as the start of EMR support from the vendor. Activation may consist of several steps: scanning charts, routing messages, managing patient flow, tracking orders, charting services and sending charges to the PMS.

Continued

Continued from previous page

Contract Issues	Issue	Typical Contract Text	Mitigation Strategy
Third Party Vendor Exclusions	EMR contracts typically exclude third party products from the obligations of the EMR vendors. The key problem is that many of these third party products were specifically selected by the EMR vendor. Although, the EMR vendor cannot vouch for all third party products, the EMR vendor should guarantee that its product will work with the specified hardware and software products that it indicates in its documentation.	Vendor is not responsible for any and all third party software or hardware products.	Practice will be provided with 12 month notice of changes to hardware and software standards for the EMR. The EMR vendor should insure that third-party software needed to support functionality of the EMR will continue to work with the EMR.
Users	A number of products are licensed by user. Users may be defined as someone on the system at any given time or on a workstation with EMR access. Users may be differentiated from those who chart patient information (e.g., doctors, nurses, PAs) and those who may access information (e.g., billing staff). Note that the definition of a user can have a substantial effect on your cost and cost comparison. For example, licensing by workstation may be more expensive that licensing by user and licensing by concurrent user. Licensing by workstation requires a license for all workstations whether they are in use or not. Similarly, licensing by user requires a license for each registered user even if not all users are using the EMR at the same time. Licensing by concurrent user requires a payment for the highest maximum number of users at any given time.	A user is anyone who accesses the software at any time.	Negotiate a reduced fee for the number of users that will be using the system. Include adequate users per provider license for vendors that license by provider. Insure that you are not paying for idle workstations and users to get the right to use the EMR.
Warranty	Many vendors fail to warrant the system, software, services or hardware. Vendors typically back off of any warranty for a variety of reasons including risk, payment and financial reporting (e.g., Sarbanes-Oxley). A practice can get caught when a vendor fails to perform but the practice is committed to continuing use of the EMR due to the difficulty of changing EMR systems.	Vendor makes no warranties, including fitness for specific purpose, for any of the software, hardware, products or services. Practice is responsible for making all decisions on the use of the software. Vendor is not responsible for how the software is used by the practice.	Include vendor warranty that the EMR software will enable the practice to comply with the applicable HIPAA Privacy and Security Standards Allow the practice to use the relevant HIPAA Transaction Sets. Insure vendor warrants that the software will support the practice in complying with the HIPAA Privacy Standards and HIPAA Security Standards.

Continued

Continued from previous page

Contract Issues	Issue	Typical Contract Text	Mitigation Strategy
	The lack of a warranty creates a number of problems for the practice. The lack of a software warranty leaves any software problem resolution at the discretion of the vendor. Having no hardware warranty leaves little recourse in the event of performance or sizing problem with the workstations or server. Unwarranted services could result in additional expenses to pay for training or implementation support that was not done the first time. You may have to struggle with incorrect guidance and information from the vendor. One of the key challenges is establishing a warranty standard. In the absence of a standard, the practice may end up in an intractable argument on the specific way the product works in a specific situation. The contract language should allow for a standard upon which the products and services will be based. The key remedy is for the vendor to correct the problem and allow your practice to go forward. Restarting the EMR implementation or switching EMR products is a costly and time-consuming effort that you should avoid.		Verify that the Vendor will offer additional enhancements to support HIPAA Transactions that may be released under the HIPAA Transaction Set requiring EMR information. Warrant that training and support services will be provided by qualified personnel and in a professional matter. The services will comply with the system requirements and include advice, instruction and services that will be an effective way to use the system. Warrant that support services will include maintenance of the product to allow the practice to meet general industry requirements as well as advice that the practice can rely on.

Track Changes—Use a markup copy of the contract in a document file. Verify that no additional changes have been made by using the document compare feature of the word-processing program. Be sure to challenge any unexpected changes. A series of unexpected changes could create some unanticipated problems or lengthen the contracting process. For example, one contract version changed the nature of the license for the entity, but created problems with the provider count that require user licenses.

Total Agreement—Constantly check the entire agreement to insure that problems and inconsistencies are addressed. Be especially careful with attachments and appendices. For example, a negotiated payment schedule in the contract may conflict with the purchase order attachment. In another case, the contract referenced Terms and Conditions on the Website that completely invalidated the negotiated terms and conditions. Consistency is especially important since the staff that administers the contract is frequently not the sales staff. ***ALERT:*** Note that the EMR accounts payable department may base their billing on the standard contract when you have negotiated alternative payment terms. A consistent contract will effectively communicate your needs and expectations. For example, one contract included the original wording for support payments in one place and a negotiated change in another. The vendor's billing department took months to determine the correct billing and render a correct bill.

Once you have completed the contract, perform a final reading to verify that the contract and attachments are correct. Once you have completed the final reading, make sure that the reviewed document is the contract that you sign. With the best of intentions, there have been mix-ups at the final signing when vendor staff used an older contract version to print the contract for signature.

LIVING WITH THE FINAL AGREEMENT

Once you have signed the contract, your still need to insure that the project proceeds according to the contract. Deviations occur for a number of reasons, including the vendor going by the standard (and *not* your negotiated) contract, and billing errors. For example . . .

> **EXAMPLE**: A project was seriously delayed due to the failure to transition from the contract to implementation on a timely basis. The contract included a timeline that was not communicated to the implementation staff.

> **EXAMPLE**: One vendor issued a combined bill for the hardware, software and support upon delivery, when the contract clearly stated that the support fees did not have to be paid until go live.

> **EXAMPLE**: A vendor rendered a bill for an upgrade to the new product version when the upgrade was included in the negotiated contract.

> **EXAMPLE**: A change order upgrade included language that superseded the original agreement.

> **EXAMPLE**: An "updated" final contract was submitted for signature that didn't include any of the agreed-upon changes.

To insure that you get the full benefits of your negotiated agreements, the contract should be the starting point for the development of supporting materials for your EMR implementation project. Transition to the implementation effort by using the negotiated agreement for the following transition tasks:

- Meet with the vendor sales and implementation team toward the end of contract negotiations or immediately after contract signing to properly structure the project and insure that all participants understand the relevant issues of the negotiated contract.

- Create a contract abstract of key information and terms as a reference tool for the project. In situations where the standard contract is supplemented by an appendix or addendum, ensure that you note the affected standard terms in the standard contract with a reference to the appendix change.

- When you compile your implementation plan, include key dates from the contract and any key issues that may effect the implementation.

The completed contract and agreement for the purchase of your EMR should be used to establish a results-oriented relationship with your EMR vendor. Your practice will have a tool to guide your implementation effort as well as structure an effective working relationship with your EMR vendor long after your have completed the initial EMR implementation.

Implementing an EMR

To guide and manage your implementation effort, you need a plan and a workflow design. Practices that do not plan ahead will be working on the fly and may make a number of decisions that will doom the project to failure or, worst yet, succeed in the implementation but fail in the clinic. For example, many practices do not set up the computerized chart to facilitate access to the chart contents. Other practices only partially implement the EMR and end up with a hybrid system that is more difficult to use. For example, a number of practices have an EMR that is used by a few doctors, but the rest of the doctors use the paper chart. Such practices must spend additional monies to maintain both methods and exchange information between the paper chart and EMR. In another situation, the EMR was used by doctors for messaging, but the paper chart was used for everything else. Such a strategy could lead to confusion and complicate maintaining the HIPAA mandated designated record set.

Vendors commonly include "project management services" in their purchase orders. What many vendors mean by project management, and what you mean/need are often very different. Typically, vendor project management services include working with your project manager on the implementation of the system. The vendor project manager will coordinate the vendor's services, keep in touch with the vendor's hardware and technical people and act as your contact point for the project. Vendor project managers will not normally manage your internal resources, third party suppliers of hardware and communications, or make decisions about how the EMR will be used in the practice. Indeed, vendors typically defer decisions to the practice which may not be in a position to make key decisions since they have never used an EMR.

Some vendors have implementation plans that describe their responsibilities but do not necessarily guide a practice through implementation. For example, one detailed vendor implementation plan had detailed step by step tasks for the vendor effort but trivialized the practice's responsibilities (e.g., practice will set up master templates). Such documents do not adequately define the scope of the project for the practice or properly quantify the practice staff and resources that will be needed to successfully deploy and activate the EMR.

Practice items are normally more numerous and complex than the EMR vendor's plan. For example, upgrading various workstations may be the responsibility of the current hardware vendor, and coordinated by your practice. Your practice may be facing a number of policy, staffing and workflow decisions that will require substantial study and research. For example, the practice may need to establish a standard for charting selected patient conditions as well as a mechanism to insure that the doctors are using the mechanism. Otherwise, the practice may not be able to determine and measure their compliance with pay for performance standards. Dealing with the current medical record requires detailed analysis of the current records and discussions with doctors that vendors may not support. For example, the doctors will need to decide on the electronic "tabs" that will be used to organize the EMR contents.

If you are using a PMS interface, your practice will be responsible for buying and installing the PMS interface as well as organizing testing between the EMR and PMS. The EMR vendor may limit its responsibilities to the receipt of PMS data. You may find it difficult to adjudicate communications and performance problems with the EMR and PMS interfaces. The EMR vendor may only focus on when the practice will be ready for training, but not necessarily the various tasks that are needed to prepare your network for the installation of the EMR server. For example, establishing work priority and the appropriate codes to flag users may require a detailed analysis of current issues and clinical practices.

Understanding practice implementation responsibilities is especially significant since the EMR vendor does not make EMR setup decisions: **your practice will need to decide how and when the EMR will be used**. You may have someone who can make these decisions or you may use a third party to help you through the process (consultant, e.g.). In either case, your project manager will be the point person for the project. In the final analysis, the EMR vendor project manager is one resource available to your practice but few vendors provide the project leadership needed to complete EMR implementation.

Dozens of strategies may be used to structure the EMR implementation. This chapter structures the EMR implementation into the following areas (Table 9.1):

CLINICAL STANDARDS

The clinical record setup defines how the EMR will be used. Clinical record setup includes practice preferences, information choices and display options. Many vendors like to point out that EMRs allow each physician to record whatever information they want

TABLE 9.1

Area	General Tasks	Resource Types	Time Frame
Clinical Standards	Establish Clinical Standards Strategy	CMO Doctors Clinical staff	Start immediately and work throughout the project.
Policy	Establish practice policies to support the EMR. Assure compliance with HIPAA and other regulatory standards. Provide a practice governance structure to support and advance EMR implementation.	Practice Management Project Manager	Mostly at beginning of project.
Project Management	Track Progress Manage Project Plan and Resources Make Decisions on Issues Address Contract Issues Resolve Problems and Issues	Project Manager Practice Manager Physician EMR Champion	Throughout the project.
Workflow and Procedures	Develop EMR Workflow Identify Use and Setup Issues to Support Workflow	Department Supervisor CMO	Created early in the project and updated as needed.
Facilities Management	Establish Secure Computer Room Adjust Offices to Accommodate EMR	Contractors	Start of Project
Technology Base	Manage Server Installation Identify Changes to Existing Hardware Identify Changes to Existing Communications Select Tablets and Other Hardware Verify Installation	Technical Support Hardware Vendors	Heavy at beginning of the project.
Software Setup	Translate Workflow Concepts to the EMR Make Setup Decisions Verify Clinical Content Develop Interface with PMS Develop Interface with Diagnostic Equipment	EMR Project Team Key Clinical Users	After Hardware Installation and Before End-User Training
Data Conversion	Develop a Scanning and Information Retrieval/Entry Strategy for Paper Charts Execute the Scanning Strategy Execute the Retrieval of Required Information from the Paper Chart and Entry into the EMR Convert data from PMS	Medical Record Staff Clinical Staff Technical Support PMS Vendor Hardware Vendor	Through EMR Go Live date
Training	Setup Training Plan Identify Training Packages Train Super Users Develop Focused Training Materials Train Staff	EMR Project Team Practice Super Users	From hardware installation to Go Live
Continuing Support	Transition to Supporting the EMR on a Day to Day Basis Establish a Maintenance Strategy	EMR Project Team	From Go Live Onward

regardless of what other physicians are doing. In the paper world, this situation is analogous to having a different intake form and/or unique clinical flow-sheet for each doctor in the practice, even if they are providing the same services. The staff has to adjust to each form and the process for each doctor. Although an EMR does not technically eliminate these differences, the practice needs to discuss the implications of these differences, and what, if any, value the differences bring to patient service, physician effectiveness, practice operations and practice performance.

In an EMR, different clinical setups and documentation standards have several implications:

Implementation Costs—If each doctor creates a different solution to the same problem, then the practice will absorb the cost of setting up the system multiple ways for the same clinical purpose. For example, some practices invest time and resources to change the order of EMR template items to match the current paper form or the preferences of one or more doctors. The practice will have to maintain multiple setups or templates for the same chief complaint or problem. As important, the doctors will each have to take their time to design the specific screens that they want. A single clinical standard will allow one doctor to work on the standard that will be used by several doctors. A single standard will *cost less* to maintain and setup.

Workflow Differences—In some cases, the clinical content reflects and/or dictates the flow of patients and issues in the practice. Different clinical chart standards may require different clinical workflows. For example, serious issues could be flagged in one manner by one doctor and another doctor may expect staff to note problems through the use of key words. The diversity of workflows could cause differences in a variety of setups and EMR uses. For example, one doctor may use a task feature to manage patient services while another doctor may use a chart note which is more difficult to manage for workflow purposes. A single standard will lead to shared workflows and enable the practice managers to use the EMR to track performance on an hourly or daily basis. For example, EMRs with workflow tools may allow the manager to quickly identify patients that have been waiting for a return call on an urgent clinical matter past a certain time limit.

Clinical Documentation—The use of different standards and rating scales could complicate the use of the EMR among the doctors and staff. Although the lack of consistency is common in paper medical records, EMRs offer more flexibility in operations by allowing many staff members to view a medical record instantaneously. By having to adjust to different reporting and documentation standards, the staff may not be as efficient. For example, one doctor may use a number to flag serious issues while another doctor may use a text note. Staff would have to be trained on the different documentation methods for each doctor.

Reporting Limitations—Using different measures, standards and record structures may complicate your ability to produce reports. For example, different doctors may use different scales, data items or information to classify patient conditions and status. Reporting would be complicated since the different scales and strategies would require complex normalization programming to produce summary statistics, or list patients with a specific condition. For example, two physicians may use different sets of adjectives to describe the same situation. The report options would have to be programmed to insure that "High" for one doctor is the same as 8 to 10 for another doctor, and "Severe" for a third doctor. The reporting situation may be further complicated when different doctors collect information that is not easily related in the EMR. For example, one doctor may collect three pieces of information that are summarized in another doctor's chart note. Complicated programming will be needed for a report containing patients from both doctors that meet a certain selection criteria. Reporting limitations are especially significant for practices that are facing pay for performance standards. If a practice cannot easily and reliably identify patients requiring a service, at risk, or with an outstanding treatment program, then the practice will not be able to effectively allocate clinical and administrative resources to ensure that patients are managed within pay for performance guidelines.

Support Costs—Maintaining the EMR clinical content and training staff will be more expensive with multiple standards for a single clinical condition. If a change is required for a clinical standard, that change would have to be programmed for each template and reported separately. Your support investment will produce a better return by focusing on refinements that allow the practice to capitalize on economies of scale instead of paying multiple times to solve the same problem in each template.

Many doctors are concerned with the loss of independence and the inability to customize their clinical records. For example, a patient chief complaint may not fit in a checklist designed by the vendor or practice. Similarly, the EMR may not allow for the textual richness that the physician uses to describe a patient condition. However, most EMR products allow physicians to insert an ad hoc note into the clinical record. Judicious use of specific notes and appropriate clinical standards will allow most practices to maintain a balance between the benefits of clinical standards and documenting unusual situations.

TIP: If the practice decides to use a single clinical standard for each clinical condition, the physicians and medical practices committee should set up a process to insure that the standard is used and evolves to meet the changing needs of the patients and physicians. The development process should include a review by the doctors that addresses the specific documentation needs of each physician and meets patient service objectives. In these situations, each change should be analyzed and reviewed to insure that the continuity of the medical record information is preserved and that the practice workflow is modified to take advantage of the change. Otherwise, the practice could encounter serious problems analyzing clinical results for pay for performance if different documentation protocols are used in a span of time.

POLICIES

Under appropriate practice governance, the practice management team needs to establish policies to support the EMR implementation and its use.

Although a number of factors will affect the particular policies you choose, one of the more challenging issues is managing and maintaining the "Designated Record Set." The HIPAA Privacy Standard defined the designated record set as:

(1) A group of records maintained by or for a covered entity that is:
  (i) The medical records and billing records about individuals maintained by or for a covered health care provider;
  (ii) The enrollment, payment, claims adjudication, and case or medical management record systems maintained by or for a health plan; or
  (iii) Used, in whole or in part, by or for the covered entity to make decisions about individuals.
(2) For purposes of this paragraph, the term *record* means any item, collection, or grouping of information that includes protected health information and is maintained, collected, used, or disseminated by or for a covered entity.

The designated record set affects your policies, transition strategy and support. The implications of the designated record set are extensive since you will be completely changing the nature, composition and usage of your medical information from a paper chart to the EMR.

Practices that include several entities (e.g., practice, therapy center, pain center and ASC) will face a challenge maintaining an individual medical record for each entity. The EMR setup, as well as the EMR features, will affect your ability to meet these requirements. For example, the EMR audit and security features may allow you to maintain separate records in the system but the separate records may be difficult to access across the entities. If you have one database for the practice and another database for the therapy center, then you will need to have a mechanism to communicate information from the clinic to the therapy center and vice versa. Otherwise, you could be in the ironic situation where the staff prints out information from the ASC's EMR to scan into the practice EMR.

The EMR implementation effort must address the transition from a paper-based medical record to an EMR. These policies help you manage patient treatment continuity and maintain the contents of the paper chart as part of your designated record set. Your practice policies must be maintained to govern the transition while making sure that you comply with the HIPAA standards. See additional information on medical record composition issues in other sections of this chapter.

Additional policy issues include:

EMR Project Management—The implementation of an EMR will affect all employees, doctors and aspects of the practice. The practice management should establish enabling policies and support for the EMR. Such policies should include support for the project and project team as well as an escalation policy to get management involved in resolving any problems. For example, an approved workflow strategy to establish a triage line for patients must be backed up by management support for the change to insure that the service is used and that individuals will not be able to bypass the practice's decision. The EMR project must have adequate resources and management support to achieve the goals of the project within the timeline established and approved by practice management.

EMR Clinical Content Management—The practice needs to formally empower the EMR Implementation Team to establish the appropriate clinical standards for the practice and implement the EMR features to support those standards. In many cases, practice clinical standards are a foreign concept. The lack of standards do not necessarily affect the other doctors in the practice. For example, the use of different intake sheet for the same condition may not be a factor if doctors typically do not collaborate on patient care. However, with the EMR, the lack of standards could inhibit the ability of the practice to capitalize on the EMR for workflow improvement, compliance, treatment management and patient care. For example, differences in EMR documentation could inhibit tracking of outstanding patient care plans and tasks. In the final analysis, the doctors are the key to clinical content management. However, the EMR Project Team needs to establish a process that guides the doctors through the approval process and insures that the doctor's decisions are implemented on a consistent basis throughout the practice. The responsibility rests with the doctors to develop a standard within the EMR and set up the EMR to take advantage of the standard. This effort may include a comprehensive analysis of the EMR clinical content, identification of issues based on the practice's needs, and development of solutions to any clinical problems or issues. The solutions should be vigorously tested and then rolled out to the clinical staff and doctors in a standardized fashion.

Establish Privacy and Security Officers—The HIPAA Privacy and Security Standards require the appointment of a Privacy Officer and a Security Officer for covered entities. If your practice is a covered entity, the EMR will dramatically empower these positions to comply with the HIPAA requirements. For example, role-based security in an EMR will allow you to comply with the HIPAA Privacy requirements. The audit trail will allow you to monitor medical record access and track disclosures. However, these features must be backed up with policies and procedures that insure timely review as well as supporting personnel policies to assure compliance. For example, the existence of an audit trail is ineffective unless the Privacy and Security Officers check for compliance with practice standards and compliance is reported to management on a periodic basis.

Audit Policies—Most EMR systems maintain audit trails of medical record changes, additions and accesses. The practice should establish audit and access policies to guide the enforcement and tracking mechanisms. The audit policies will determine when the audit trails will be analyzed and where the audit will focus. Audit focus may be driven by policy changes or previous analysis of audit issues. For example, you may conduct periodic audit trail review of medical record for patients in the public eye that is backed up by stringent personnel policies. Note that audit reports to management should be based on a reporting period and not purely driven by exceptions and problems.

Security Policies—Security policies should address the physical, administrative and technical security safeguards mandated by the HIPAA Security Standards. The policies should recognize a security standard for the practice, as well as a process to review security issues and vulnerabilities on a periodic basis. You could let incidents trigger a security review (e.g., hardware changes or software installation), or conduct the reviews every six months or once annually. Security policies should cover a wide range of issues including the maintenance of offsite backups, backup standards, computer room access, authorization standards for doctors and employees, training standards and reporting protocols. The security policies should also include an appropriate report to the Security Officer and practice management on the current compliance status of the practice. This way the practice will meet the HIPAA requirements as well as maintain appropriate controls over the EMR system and data. This process should include items that may be "behind the scenes" of your system, such as firewalls, virus software and general access to your computer systems. Indeed, many problems can be traced back to a series of violations that lead to a significant problem. For more information on HIPAA Security Standards, contact the Office of HIPAA Standards at CMS.

Notice of Privacy Practices—The HIPAA Privacy standards mandate that covered entities have a Notice of Privacy Practices. A new consent or acknowledgement of the notice is required for any substantive changes to the Notice of Privacy Practices. The Notice of Privacy Practices may require changes to accommodate the EMR. For example, the EMR may affect the tracking of disclosures, availability of medical records and nature of medical records that can be provided to the patient. The practice should consult with legal counsel to determine if the current Notice of Privacy Practices will require changes to accommodate the EMR. In any event, your EMR will effect how you manage privacy issues and meet the release of information needs of patients. Note that you need to verify that privacy information is easily accessible to EMR users to assure compliance with patient limitations and issues. For example, some EMRs allow for an alert message that is displayed when a patient record is accessed. You could note any privacy issues on the alert message.

Personal Use—An EMR significantly increases the risk of loss from a system failure or problem. Practice policies may be created to significantly limit or prohibit the personal use of practice computers. Personal computer use has exposed practices to viruses and other damaging corruptions. For example, downloading freeware into a practice-based computer exposed a network of 100 workstations to a 2-day stoppage due to a virus that overloaded the mail server. In other cases, loading a game onto a workstation created a conflict with critical software needed to run the EMR. The more control you assert over system use, the less chance of a problem for your system.

Clinical Data Access—When an employee looks at a paper chart, the paper chart does not make a record of the access. An EMR allows instantaneous access to any medical record subject to security constraints. Some EMRs allow you to limit access by type of clinical information, and even to a list of selected patients. Depending on the capability of your EMR, you may be able to limit EMR access based on patient type, location and a number of other options. However, the EMR makes a record of every employee action for future reference and review. The practice may want to define a specific policy and review standard to limit employee access to the need-to-know standard of the HIPAA Privacy Standards. Such a process should consider the retention strategy for these access logs. For example, you will want to keep adequate logs online to look back and review problems even though such logs may consume a fair amount of disk space. In some cases, these policies may affect other relationships. For example, one practice could not dismiss employees for inappropriate access to the medical records due to a union agreement.

Role-Based Access—The HIPAA Privacy Standards require the use of a role-based access strategy. Ideally, the practice should design and establish an access policy based on the definition of roles. Each role would have a defined access and edit capability. The policy should allow for exceptions to be approved by the Security and/or Privacy Officer with appropriate reporting to practice management. Note that exceptions to the role-based security strategy should be reviewed and approved by appropriate practice supervisors and/or management. For example, some EMRs allow the user to violate security access in an emergency. Typically, the EMR records the unauthorized access in a special audit log. However, someone needs to check the log to verify the emergency access.

Paper Record Retention—Practices pursuing paperless medical records will need paper retention policies to support the EMR. A paper retention policy will be needed for existing paper charts that are scanned into the EMR as well as paper documents received from the Go Live date going forward. The paper retention policy should be developed in consultation with your legal counsel and malpractice insurance carrier. For example, your legal counsel may not have a problem shredding the documents when scanned, but your malpractice carrier may require retention for a year. For example, some states recognize the EMR chart as a valid and legal replacement for the paper chart from the day the EMR chart is available. Typically, the paper charts are retained for a certain period after scanning of the chart. Miscellaneous paper documents scanned after EMR Go Live are typically retained for a certain period after the document is scanned. Note that some practices shred the charts and paper documents as soon as the information is scanned. If you keep the documents, make sure that you have a strategy to locate a document in the unlikely event that you need to get the original. For example, you may file the scanned documents by date and user.

Implementation Policies—EMR implementation is a strategic move by a practice. Practices need to consider what, if any inducements or penalties will be used to insure that the EMR is adopted by the physicians and employees. If some physicians are using the EMR, and others are not, then the practice will have to maintain the paper records as well as pay for the EMR. Some physician practices establish policies that insure the paper records will be eliminated. For example, the EMR implementation is based on a strict guideline and timeframe. Policy options include establishing a clinical standard for the practice and terminating availability and access to the paper records after a certain date. On the financial side, physicians who continue to use dictation and paper medical records could be charged for paper medical records and the EMR computer system in their compensation formula.

Practice policies are key tools to convey management support for the EMR implementation. The right polices will avoid a myriad of implementation challenges and insure that the EMR project is adequately supported. This way, the implementation effort can focus on a successful implementation and not get sidetracked with the question of whether the practice should have an EMR. For example, one practice implemented an EMR which was not adequately supported by management. The project went through many sudden changes and was significantly delayed.

PROJECT MANAGEMENT

Managing an EMR implementation project encompasses a number of tasks and issues. Unfortunately, few practices are fully aware of the scope of managing an EMR project due to the lack of clarity in the EMR vendor relationship. Typically, vendors do not expand upon practice responsibilities and process. Vendor project meetings frequently monitor your progress in preparing for the next vendor step, but do not necessarily specify the types of tasks you need to manage. For example, an EMR vendor may say that you need to set up the scanning system, but it will not walk you through standardizing your document descriptions, capturing scanned images or the disposition of the scanned documents.

To succeed, the practice needs to manage resources for the EMR project. Some practices use internal resources, although few practices have internal expertise in EMR implementation. Some practices use vendor resources at an additional charge, and other practices use independent consultants. Vendor EMR expertise may be offset by the independence of an external consultant. In some situations, vendor staff may not be able to act as an advocate on the practice's behalf in the event of problems and misunderstandings. For example, an error may not be as vigorously pursued by a vendor's employee. In other situations, vendor conversion errors may by corrected by the practice staff rather than the vendor redoing the work correctly.

Regardless of your strategy, the project should be guided by a formal management process as well as management tools:

> **Project Plan**—A project plan is a running list of the various EMR to-do items. The project plan is used to monitor project steps and includes administrative, technical, workflow and other implementation issues. Project plans may be managed

through a spreadsheet, project management product or a word-processing table. The project plan should be initially compiled with as much detail as possible. The actual items will evolve as the project proceeds, so you can respond and focus on evolving issues. For example, an initial project plan may specify that the current workstations need to be reviewed to meet the minimum EMR requirements. As the project proceeds, specific tasks may be defined to upgrade various workstations. **ALERT:** A basic project plan is located at the end of this chapter.

Key Issues—A variety of problems and issues will arise as the project proceeds. From getting a policy decision on record retention to scheduling staff and doctors for training, problems and issues must be tracked and managed. In some cases, the issues may affect progress and, in other cases, issues may involve evolving issues. For example, EMR reports may require review by a clinical practices committee that has yet to be formed. In another case, you may want to set up sessions with key referring practices to train them on the changes to your procedures and outgoing reports. A sample key issues table follows (see Table 9.2), and another sample can be found at the end of this chapter.

Timeline—Project plans are great tools for managing a project, but they may not be the best tools to communicate with the project team. Project plans can consist of 100s of implementation items spread across a couple dozen pages. However, most people involved in EMR implementation will not be able to understand the complete project plan or dig through the details that they need to know. You should consider supplementing the project plan with a project timeline. The project timeline presents key events and issues affecting the EMR project. While the project manager is responsible for the detailed plan and issues, the rest of the project team needs a tool to understand the context of the project and evolving issues. A timeline can focus on the more immediate issues and additional details added as the project proceeds. The timeline can be annotated with important information for the project. For example, you can highlight key critical

TABLE 9.2

Area	Issues	Status	Assigned	Start	Due	Comment

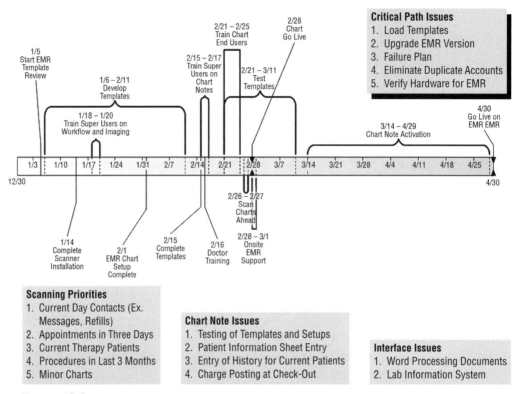

Critical Path Issues
1. Load Templates
2. Upgrade EMR Version
3. Failure Plan
4. Eliminate Duplicate Accounts
5. Verify Hardware for EMR

Scanning Priorities
1. Current Day Contacts (Ex. Messages, Refills)
2. Appointments in Three Days
3. Current Therapy Patients
4. Procedures in Last 3 Months
5. Minor Charts

Chart Note Issues
1. Testing of Templates and Setups
2. Patient Information Sheet Entry
3. Entry of History for Current Patients
4. Charge Posting at Check-Out

Interface Issues
1. Word Processing Documents
2. Lab Information System

FIGURE 9.1

path issues and important strategies. A one page document presents a concise view of the project and will help your group understand the big picture. A sample timeline is shown in Figure 9.1.

Critical Path Diagram—Another useful project management tool is the critical path plan. The critical path plan graphically shows the relationship and sequence of items by category. The critical path plan will help highlight the key tasks and status as the plan progresses. For example, the critical path plan may show the relationship between hardware installation and the start of training. A sample critical path diagram is shown in Figure 9.2.

Clinical Content Tracking—EMR projects that include clinical content changes or development should use a separate table to manage the clinical content. The clinical content items should be listed for the practice, and the various steps should be tracked and monitored. In general, clinical content efforts take the most time and require the most limited resources: doctors and clinicians. At a minimum, your staff should verify the clinical content, to define any changes and enhancements. Depending on your EMR strategy and tools, you may want to hold off on implementing any changes until you have verified that there is not a viable workaround. In the absence of an alternative handling of the clinical situation, any changes should be tested and approved by the appropriate doctors and clinicians. A sample clinical content tracking table is shown in Table 9.3.

FIGURE 9.2

A single document or tool will not help you to communicate with all of the various internal parties involved in the project. Using a combination of project plan, timelines and, if appropriate, critical path diagrams will insure that the details as well as the big picture project issues can be effectively planned, communicated and coordinated according to the various needs and interests of the EMR project team.

Possessing the tools of the project is very different from managing the project. Managing the project includes assigning tasks, organizing resources and coordinating the effort of

TABLE 9.3

Clinical Area	Assign to	Review EMR Content	Inventory Issues/ Changes	Design Changes/ Setup	Program Changes/ Setup	Unit Test Changes/ Setup	Field Test	Present to Drs/ Staff
Internal Medicine								
OB/GYN								
Cardiology								
Nurse Triage								
Advice Line								

various parties. As soon as you have chosen your product, you should identify an EMR project team for the practice. The internal project team will not necessarily include an EMR vendor representative. As a practical matter, the vendor representative should not be privy to a number of project issues including strategies for dealing with issues and managing other vendors. Additionally, the practice may need to undertake extensive discussions of policy, strategy, and operational issues that are avoided by many vendors. The project team should consist of the following resources:

Project Manager—The project manager is the guide and architect of your EMR effort. Depending on the internal resources and expertise, the project manager may be an internal or external resource. The key role of the project manager is to set expectations, track progress and address issues. The project manager will be responsible for working with internal resources to get everyone up to speed and focus efforts on the implementation effort. The project manager role should include helping the practice arrive at decisions on using the EMR as well as compelling doctors and staff to support the EMR project. Such efforts may include one-on-one discussions and dealing with key needs of a particular doctor or staff person. For example, a doctor may be concerned about how they will be able to access information that their nurses record on a log that is kept on the doctor's desk. If the EMR contains the information, the project manager may arrange for a special report or screen view to be made available to the doctor.

Technical Resource—In the final analysis, the practice will need a key person to address technical issues and problems. The EMR is too important to leave all support to an outside party. You do not necessarily want a high-level technical person, but rather someone who can work with staff on common problems and issues as well as coordinate the resolution of more complex issues with the EMR vendor or hardware vendor. Ideally, the internal person should be able to help staff address day-to-day issues and needs. For a once a month or a once a year issue, you may decide to use an outside resource such as a systems integrator or a local network management team. The technical resource should be knowledgeable of your current technology base and work with the appropriate vendors on upgrades to support the EMR.

Clinical Resource(s)—Depending on the nature and size of the practice, clinical resources may include doctors and nurses. At a minimum, clinical resources should *include a subject matter expert in each clinical area* covered by the practice. In many cases, more than one clinical resource will be needed. Primary care practices may have too broad a set of clinical areas to be managed by one person, and specialty practices may need support in sub-specialty areas. Scribes and technicians may also serve as clinical resources. Practices in which doctors do their own documentation will want to use doctors as clinical resources. The clinical resources are charged with verifying the clinical content and practice setup. They also become the defacto resident experts to the staff as the EMR is activated. Therefore, you need people who have the time, skills and will to help the other people in your practice use the EMR. The clinical resources will review the clinical content and make adjustments as needed. However, any adjustments should be carefully reviewed to determine that the adjustment is effective and appropriate as well as not already handled by the EMR. For example, some practices have developed a strategy outside of the standard product to perform a function that is built into the EMR product. The clinical resources will coordinate testing, perform training and support other implementation efforts. A key challenge will be to manage patient services while the EMR effort proceeds. The implementation schedule should allow adequate time for the doctors and other clinicians to work the EMR efforts into their schedules. You need one or more doctors who are willing to put in the time to verify that the EMR clinical content will support your practice, and spend the time to become familiar enough and confident enough to move forward with using the EMR.

Medical Records Resource—The medical records resource should be the manager or supervisor of the Medical Records Department. The medical records resource will be responsible for formulating, testing and executing the conversion strategy for paper charts as well as supporting the flow of electronic medical record information. A survey of current paper medical records as well as testing of various scanning and paper management strategies may be necessary. The paper medical record strategy and supporting policy drives this effort. However, the real challenge is the conversion of the paper records to the EMR. Depending on your go live strategy and scanning decision, the handing of the existing paper record in the conversion effort is a massive undertaking. Whether you are scanning selected pieces of the paper chart or entering key information into the EMR (Ex. Previous procedures, and immunizations), the medical records resource will need excellent management skills and be in a position to support this important aspect of the conversion effort.

Business Office Resource—The business office uses information from the EMR to justify claims as well as dispute claim payment with payers. Front desk staff will scan clinical information into the EMR and trigger the tracking of patient office flow in the EMR. The daily reconciliation process will be redesigned to reconcile charge posting from the EMR to the PMS. Additional procedures may verify task completion standards. For example, the Business Office may verify that all tasks are completed on a daily basis. Otherwise, the number of outstanding tasks will become unmanageable. The business office resource must work on insuring the continuing billing process in the absence of a paper chart and even without a fee slip. This effort may be made all the more difficult for practices that replace their PMS before implementing the EMR.

To manage the project on a daily basis, the project manager must maintain contact with the appropriate working teams to monitor progress and address issues. Several forums can be used to maintain project momentum:

Ad-Hoc Discussions—The quantity and complexity of issues is a major problem for managing an EMR project. The number and variety of issues that arise can be daunting. EMR issues could include who gets a tablet, verifying the medical record generated by the EMR, training staff and deciding on changes to clinical workflow. The parties that can resolve and address any pending issues need to have the flexibility to pull away for meetings on appropriate matters. Some practices have experienced serious delays due to scheduling issues. For example, one practice had to wait two weeks to hold a meeting with managers on medical record scanning. Flexibility and quick response to evolving EMR issues will insure that you maintain project momentum and continuity. This situation is especially challenging during the initial rollout of the EMR when adjustments may be needed on a real time basis.

Vendor Project Meetings—Most vendors use project management meetings to coordinate the vendor resources. Vendor project manager meetings frequently address the expected services and activities of the vendor in light of the current practice efforts. Typically, vendors do not see their role as making the decision on what to do, but offer the practice options on what is possible with the product. The vendor meetings may be held with the entire practice EMR project team or key representatives from your EMR project team. **TIP:** Make sure that you are prepared to take the initiative and effectively manage the vendor. In a number of cases, vendors defer to the practice on issues that the practice staff is not prepared to address. The outstanding issues can lead to delays and even additional costs. In order to avoid such problems, the practice should keep track of all issues and insure that the vendor provides an agenda for project meetings. In the absence of a comprehensive agenda, you may not be able to meet your meeting objectives or even have the practice staff needed to arrive at a decision.

Internal Project Meetings—Internal project meetings are used to coordinate the efforts of staff and monitor progress. The internal meetings may be held every week or two depending on the project stage and activities. The project meetings should be based on an agenda and notes of key decisions should be published and shared after the meeting. In some cases, project meetings will result in changes to the other project management tools. Internal project meetings should involve the entire EMR project team, but not necessarily the vendor. The internal project team may be discussing issues that are not relevant or appropriate for the vendor. In some cases, the internal project meetings may include a changing set of participants. For example, initially you may include the PMS vendor to deal with interface issues, or the manager of the first office to go live with the EMR.

The key project goal is maintaining the pace of work, and keeping the team up-to-date on evolving issues. Many EMR projects get sidetracked due to competing priorities and lack of progress. The implementation of an EMR involves a complete set of work in addition to the continuing operations of the practice. If you do not have additional resources to support the EMR effort, you risk delays in implementation or failures due to a lack of focus.

Before you proceed, make sure that you have a workable plan and you feel confident in the capabilities of the software and the project team. For example, one practice scanned more than 30,000 medical records into its EMR. After the scanning process, the practice discovered that the EMR enhancements would not work for the practice and it moved to another product. The conversion of the images from the "old" EMR was difficult due to technology problems. In another situation, an EMR project was undertaken by a single clinician without the support of the practice or staff. The goal of the project was to "try" a medical record, but the project was merely a waste of time and money.

Project plans dramatically differ among practices due the differences in the various implementation areas. For example, an EMR project that includes extensive clinical content efforts will differ from a project that takes clinical content "out of the box." To formulate the implementation plan that is right for you, consider the issues outlined in Table 9.4.

After designing the project plan, the plan should be maintained as needed to track the project and problems. The project manager should feel free to edit, delete, split and combine items to keep the plan current and useful. For example, you may have expected to develop an interface that is available from a third party. Once the go forward decision is made, the plan should be updated. Note that the practice (not the EMR vendor) EMR implementation plan can run to several dozen pages, but the use of timelines and plan summaries will help you highlight the important issues that the project team should focus on.

In the course of the EMR project, you will encounter problems. The problems may be self inflicted or a function of how certain components work together. For example, you may find that an expected interface is not available, or that the condition of the medical records precludes certain conversion strategies. In any event, you need to insure that you can get the relevant project team resources organized to address the problem, adjust the plan, and move forward.

WORKFLOW AND PROCEDURES

From the initial call on a patient problem to the office visit and follow-up tracking, the EMR will change the way you record, use and access information. How you manage and prepare for this change will affect your entire effort.

Given that these massive changes will occur, you need a strategy to practically manage, guide and deal with the EMR. Some practices wait until the system is installed to "see what happens." Other practices look to the vendor to guide the changes. If you wait until the system is installed, you may corrupt your EMR effort with constant changes. If you look to your vendor, you may not get a solution that best fits your practice. The time between signing your contract and the installation of the hardware can be used to formulate your EMR vision.

To put the issues into perspective, look at how you would go about the design of a new office. Would you go to a hardware store and buy the materials without a blueprint?

TABLE 9.4

Area	PROJECT MANAGEMENT ISSUES TO CONSIDER
General	What are the key project task areas and what are the resources needed for each area? What are the current critical path items and who is responsible for addressing them? How much time can the EMR Team members practically dedicate to the project on a daily basis? How much time can "champion" doctors practically commit to the EMR project? What addition resources will be needed and for how long?
Clinical Standards	What are the clinical content areas that require verification? What clinical content areas require substantial development? Who are the key physicians and other clinical staff in each clinical area that could work on EMR implementation? What is the verification process? What is the development and modification strategy? What is the testing strategy? What is the deployment and activation strategy?
Policy	What are the practice policies that need approval from the practice management team? What policies require legal counsel and/or risk manager advice? What policies are needed to prevent acceptance problems and issues? What is the escalation policy to insure quick resolution to problems and resistance? What is the governance structure that will represent practice management for the EMR implementation?
Project Management	What are the resources that will be available to support the EMR project? What staffing strategies will be used to maintain continuity during the project? What are the reporting and management lines for the EMR project? How often will meetings be held for the practice EMR project team? How often will management meetings be held with the vendor?
Workflow and Procedures	Who are the key people who understand current operations? What workflow packages are needed to guide the EMR project? How will workflow changes be approved and implemented? What are the organizational changes needed to support workflow changes? How will the departments be reorganized to capitalize on the EMR? What process will be used to reassign and redesign staff positions?
Facilities Management	Where can the computer room be placed? What other facility accommodations are needed for the EMR? What level of security does the practice need to reasonably reduce risks? What physical areas are available to support medical record scanning?
Technology Base	What are the current technologies that may need further review? What are the hardware investments needed to mitigate the risk of EMR failure within the practice's budget? What hardware will be support an effective server base for the EMR? What workstation and tablet models will be used by the practice? What are the scanning, and printing requirements of the various departments and locations? What verification process is needed to validate the delivery and installation of equipment? What verification process is needed to check the interoperability of system components?
Software Setup	What current information is needed to support EMR setup? How will expected changes to the practice effect EMR use? What policies are needed to support software setup? What testing is needed for interfaces to the PMS and diagnostic equipment? What is the timing of the initial download of patient demographic and appointment information into the EMR?

Area	PROJECT MANAGEMENT ISSUES TO CONSIDER
Data Conversion	What process will be used to determine the disposition of paper medical records? What resources will be needed to prepare and process information from the paper records into the EMR? What strategy will be used for converting existing electronic data to the EMR? What hardware, facility and staffing resources will be needed to support the EMR? How will the data conversion process assure quality and avoid duplication of information?
Training	What training materials will be needed to support the project? How will the practice train doctors and support doctors in their initial use of the EMR? What training tasks will be done by practice staff? How will training be broken down into manageable pieces for users? How will super-user training differ from regular-user training? What materials will be needed to deal with cross-vendor training related to hardware and interfaces? What supplemental training plans will be used to develop staff knowledge and flexibility?

Would you leave the design decisions to the construction crew? The approach of most practices to EMR implementation is analogous to building an office without an architect or a general contractor. One way to avoid such a problem is to develop a workflow model that will serve as your blueprint for the EMR implementation.

The workflow effort will help you cope with the real effects of an EMR. Key changes to consider include:

Staff Interactions and Use—EMRs with workflow features will enable staff to interact on patient service issues. The workflow model supports the entry and tracking of patient tasks. For example, a task can be sent to a doctor on a patient issue and forwarded to another staff person for follow-up. The EMR simplifies the use of staff by physicians and provides a tracking tool to manage patient issues. As important, an alternative view of the pending tasks will help supervisors identify problems and proactively address patient needs.

Instantaneous Access—EMR supports immediate access to patient medical records. EMRs eliminate the problems with co-locating patient issues, the medical chart and the provider. For example, some practices use a message center or phone message service to take patient messages with the prospect of a return call to the patient. If the EMR provides instantaneous access, should your practice have a nurse line and address specific problems immediately? For those practices with nurse lines, the EMR will empower the nurses to more effectively address and document patient issues. Indeed, you may be able to address a patient issue during the call. Such a response will reduce patient anxiety and make better use of staff and doctors. Thereby, doctors could have more time to deal with the more serious issues and problems.

Information Velocity—By storing and routing images, lab results, faxes and other items, EMRs significantly speed up the flow of information. For example, an interfaced diagnostic test may cut several steps from patient test ordering and results access. The speed could change the way the practice manages patient services as well as how staff coordinates care with the doctors. For example, an EMR interface with a diagnostic tool cut intake processing time in half for a specialty practice. The faster intake cut wait times and resulted in less wait time for the doctors and patients. As important, you may be able to server more patients with the same diagnostic equipment.

Before you start considering the effect of the changes and set up your workflow "blueprint," gather some important information on your current status and the tools you will be working with:

Cataloging Current Clinical Data—Some practices have no clinical forms and do everything in free form notes, and/or transcription. Other practices have a wide range of clinical documentation tools and forms. Intake forms, clinical forms and treatment plans are examples of existing clinical data.

Initially, the practice should gather copies of every form used in the clinical areas. Clinical forms may include patient intake forms, check-off sheets for specific diseases or chief complaints, order forms for services and therapy and surgery scheduling request documents. **TIP**: If you have multiple offices or departments, make sure that your get copies of the different forms used at different locations and even forms used by different doctors.

For each form, you should document the source of the form, situations the form is used for and the relevant staff or doctors. You should carefully note any special or unclear information on the form as well as any special usage issues. For example, a form may include a coding system that is unique to the doctor. In some situations, the practice may use the form for a unique case, perhaps because there is no other form available or the form has never been updated.

Document Current Procedures—To get a clear picture of your situation, review your current procedures. Current procedures may be documented in a manual, written notes held by staff members or other informal documentation. The current procedure documentation will facilitate the design of new procedures and workflow with the EMR.

If you have a current procedure manual, the manual should be verified with the actual office operation. The procedure review process should identify the actual procedures that are used as well as key nuances and exceptions. Even if you have a procedures manual, verify the current procedures and clinical processes.

Some practices have no written procedures and rely on a key person or the staff to know how to function. However, the HIPAA standards require a written procedure that establishes the operational standard for the practice. At the end of the EMR implementation process, you will be well positioned to create such a document. However, you will need current procedure information to guide the EMR project. In these cases, you should invest the time briefly to document the current procedures. The documentation does not have to be formal, but the information is necessary to guide your EMR workflow design process.

In either case, the practice should gather information on the actual patient service and clinical management processes. Be especially careful to document hand-offs among staff and doctors as well as the information that is communicated among the various departments. For example, some procedure manuals mention the doctor passing the patient onto diagnostic services, when the patient actually was served by diagnostic services at the direction of mid-level staff. These details will guide the EMR team in designing the workflow that establishes the use of the software and the assignment of hardware to staff.

Include the nuances that will be significant to the EMR project. For example, some locations may use different procedures since they offer other services, feature other staff or have unique equipment. In some cases, different procedures are not based on any clinical or organizational issue; no one ever tried to standardize procedures across all locations.

Compile a List of Key EMR Features—A list of key EMR features will help you determine the effect of the EMR on your processes. The key features can be derived from the EMR analysis. Key features include scanning, tasking, templates, clinical orders, clinical content and patient routing. Surgical scheduling, transcription and patient surveys should also be documented. The key features document should include a few brief observations on the feature, as well as the general implications of the feature for the practice. You may even include a screen sample to clarify the EMR option. For **EXAMPLE**,

> A description can be assigned to a scanned image. The user, date and time are automatically assigned to the scanned image. The description should be structured to consistently identify the key image information.
>
> Tasks may have a due date and priority that can affect clinical standards. Performance standards may be established for responding to tasks with a certain priority. A management function may be established to monitor overdue tasks as well as retrospectively analyze performance and response.
>
> Patient flow may be tracked through the appointment schedule that notes patient status and location. The practice standards would define when the status or location is changed and the significance of status codes.

The information on current clinical issues and the product highlights are your reference point for the development of a new workflow model. After gathering the current information, you should consider establishing the optimal workflow model for the practice. You may be wondering how you can create a new model without getting specific EMR training. However, you should have a general idea of what the system does from your decision-making process. After compiling a list of requirements, attending demonstrations, analyzing various products and visiting a site, you should have a good idea of what the EMR can do for you. If necessary, conduct another demonstration with the vendor as a kick-off to you effort. The next question to answer is how the EMR should operate in your practice.

The workflow design itemizes your expectations and vision. This document will be a blueprint or reference point for the rest of your effort. Thereby, you have a tool to guide you in working with the vendor as well as help you evaluate the effect of various decisions and strategies on your practice. Without such a tool, you will be constantly reacting to the collateral effects of every change and issue. The workflow strategy allows you to look at the situation and issues before your get absorbed in the intensity of EMR implementation. Practices that make it up as they go along frequently end up with partial EMR implementations that do not fully capitalize on their EMR investment.

In support of your workflow design, you need a workflow design facilitator. The facilitator can be an internal or external resource. External facilitators may be useful since they are not tied to your current problems and processes. External facilitators may also have experience implementing EMRs and knowledge of technical issues that may be lacking in your practice. An internal facilitator may be useful since they have a deep understanding of your operation and patients. You may also consider EMR vendor facilitators. However, many EMR vendors do not provide such services and some vendors may impose a model that is not the best solution for your practice. A non-vendor facilitator will help you explore all of your options and help you think creatively. For example, one vendor facilitator tried to impose an operational model that was successful in an orthopedic practice on an ophthalmology practice with an optical shop. The handoff to the optical shop was not fully developed and the shop was not fully integrated into the EMR. The optical shop continued to use its paper-based forms and logs outside of the EMR. Therefore, the optical shop staff was recording prescription information on a form that printed by their EMR system in the same office.

You can document the workflow in several different formats. You can document the workflow using written procedures and/or a flowchart (see below). The purpose of the workflow design is not to document every keystroke and patient interaction. **The workflow design should define the movement and handling of information in the practice.** You can start with general workflow concepts and add details as you proceed. Going forward, you will catalog issues that you uncover, key system features that will be used and setup requirements. See the example on the next page.

Documenting the key EMR functions needed for the relevant area will help you plan training as well as insure that you consider all of the effected areas when you design your EMR setup. For example, immunization order tracking and fulfillment may affect patient scheduling, patient intake and patient routing in a pediatric practice. A pediatric practice would want immunizations to be considered in the patient routing steps and orders as well as the recall strategy (see Figure 9.3).

To work with manageable areas, break the workflow into the various areas of your practice. The workflow documentation will become the basis for the setup of the EMR, your

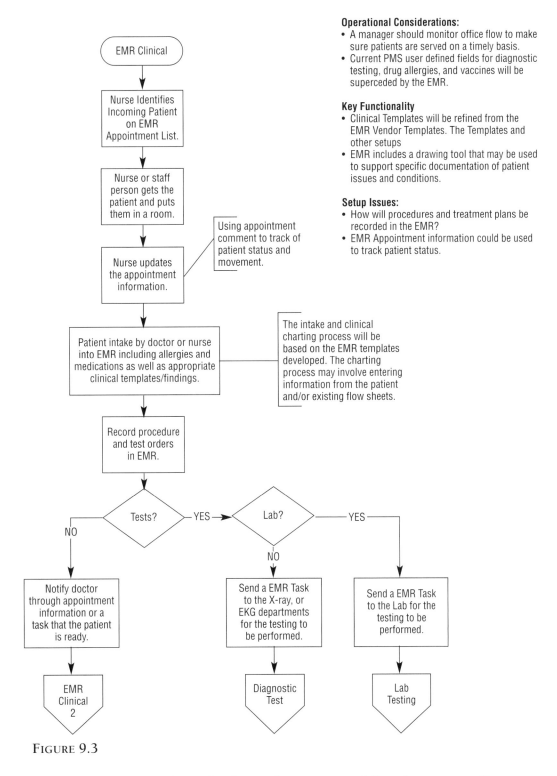

Operational Considerations:
• A manager should monitor office flow to make sure patients are served on a timely basis.
• Current PMS user defined fields for diagnostic testing, drug allergies, and vaccines will be superceded by the EMR.

Key Functionality
• Clinical Templates will be refined from the EMR Vendor Templates. The Templates and other setups
• EMR includes a drawing tool that may be used to support specific documentation of patient issues and conditions.

Setup Issues:
• How will procedures and treatment plans be recorded in the EMR?
• EMR Appointment information could be used to track patient status.

FIGURE 9.3

detailed procedures and even hardware placement. Workflow design even affects your training plan and strategy. The following table gives you some issues to consider in your workflow effort (see Table 9.5).

TABLE 9.5

Area	WORKFLOW ISSUES TO CONSIDER
General	What overlapping functionality exists in the EMR and PMS systems? Which product (EMR or PMS) will be relied upon to address the overlapping issues? What are the key features of the EMR that should be considered in the new workflow? How does the EMR impact the allocation of employees to the various practice areas and locations? How can the EMR improve the organization of the practice by modality, doctor, pod and/or department? How will the velocity of information flow affect the working styles and workload of clinical staff and doctors? Where does the EMR effect the utilization of administrative staff by clinical operations?
Appointment Scheduling	How can the appointment scheduler access information on pending patient services to more effectively schedule appointments? How can the appointment scheduler track expected test results in working with patients on upcoming visits? What connection is maintained between outstanding services, recalls and appointment scheduling?
Medical Records	What are the scanning strategies and standards for the current paper chart? What events will trigger the scanning of the patient's paper chart into the EMR? What are the response requirements for chart-scanning tasks? How will Medical Records prioritize scanning of charts for same day visits, as well as messages, prescription refills and other priorities? How will scanned patient charts be indicated in the EMR and PMS? How will Medical Records produce outgoing medical information including referral letters and medical record releases? How will Medical Records maintain disclosure logs in the EMR? How will release of information requests be logged and tracked in the EMR? How will ROI activities and disclosures be logged in the EMR?
Phone Triage	What are the priorities for the various phone messages received by the practice? What are the treatment and clinical advice guidelines for patients calling in for service or advice? What is the routing strategy by message types to the appropriate clinical staff? What routing options could the practice use to make better use of clinical resources? How does message routing affect clinical staff utilization? What are the escalation strategies that are possible with the EMR? How will non-patient messages be managed? Should a central call center be used by the practice? What performance tracking measures will the practice want to use for phone triage calls?
Check-In	What PMS based information is needed in the EMR? How will the information be recorded in the EMR? What will be done with clinical documents delivered to the check-in desk by the patient? How will the information be routed? How will the appropriate clinical staff be notified? How will the clinical area be notified of patient arrivals through the EMR? What patient clinical information will be captured at check-in? How? What is the assumption/requirement for information transfer from the PMS to the EMR for clinical treatment?
Initial Intake	How does the EMR effect the assignment of intake staff to doctors and patients? What information should be gathered at intake to smooth the clinical process? To what extent should pending patient orders be managed at patient intake? How will the intake staff identify patients ready for service? What documentation requirements will be fulfilled at the initial intake? What services should be performed or triggered before the patient is seen by the doctor? What, if any, historical data should be entered into the EMR during the first patient visit after EMR Go Live? What are the care triggers to enter historical clinical information into a patient's record? How will the intake staff notify the clinical staff on the patient status?

Area	WORKFLOW ISSUES TO CONSIDER
Clinical Treatment	What is the effect of the EMR on the departmental organization of the clinical areas? What is the workflow standard for clinical services in the practice? What clinical workflow variations are needed to accommodate subspecialties or location (e.g., equipment, services) differences? What are the doctor sign-off standards for patient services provided by mid-level staff? How should additional services be verified for payer coverage and/or referral requirements? Does the process affect the entry of an order into the EMR? How are orders for ancillary, lab and diagnostic services recorded and communicated to the appropriate department? What are the treatment plans and follow-up standards for key clinical conditions? Where and how will prescriptions be presented to the patient? Where and how will patient education be presented to the patient? Where and how will information on procedures be presented to the patient? How are follow-up treatment plan items recorded and managed? What is the time line for treatment plans prescribed by the doctors?
Diagnostic Studies	How will the technicians track pending study orders? What process will be used to assimilate the diagnostic images into the EMR? How will the EMR be used to track the status of diagnostic studies: ordered, completed, reviewed and accepted? What is the routing protocol for diagnostic study orders? What are the performance tolerances for diagnostic studies?
Lab	How will the lab track pending lab orders? How is the performing lab selected for a patient? How will EMR lab orders be entered into the Lab Information System? What mechanism will transfer the lab results to the EMR?
Ancillary Services	What are the priorities for services and how are those priorities indicated? How can the practice smooth the conversion of the patient from the clinic to ancillary services? How are ancillary service orders managed? What status information should be maintained for patients receiving ancillary services? What documentation standards should be used to simplify the reporting of patient status to the doctor? How are product orders (e.g., DME, hearing aids, contacts) managed and tracked?
Check-Out	Is there any EMR information that needs to be reflected in the PMS? How? What, if any, editing of charges from the EMR will be necessary before posting to the PMS? What can the check-out staff do to charge information from the EMR?
Transcription	How does the EMR track dictation that is to be added to the patient's EMR record? How will transcription tasks be tracked in the practice? What effect does the EMR have on outside transcription services? How long will transcription support continue? How will the EMR support the review and distribution of transcribed documents?
Surgery Scheduling	How will the surgical scheduler be informed of pending patient surgeries? How will the surgery scheduler manage the various clinical and administrative issues associated with surgery scheduling? Where will the patient forms and information print for the patient? What status information on pending surgeries will be available to practice staff and doctors? Where will signed patient forms be kept and how will the forms be organized? What information will be saved in the PMS and EMR? How will the information in the two systems be kept current?

Area	WORKFLOW ISSUES TO CONSIDER
Billing	How will posted charges be reconciled between the EMR and PMS systems? What process will verify the coding of charges? How will coded changes be reflected in the EMR? How will the billing department identify PMS claims requiring EMR documentation? Where will the billing department locate and access reports and documentation needed for claims submission?
Recall	What recall standards will be established for key diseases and conditions? How will recalls information be coordinated between the EMR and PMS?
Collections	What EMR information does the payer collections staff need access to? What format and information will be generated from the EMR system to substantiate submitted claims? What are the transmission options and standards for sending clinical information from the EMR to the payer?
Incoming Documents	How will incoming faxes and other incoming documents be added to the patient medical record? What tools are available to support physician signoff and management of incoming documents? What is the routing protocol for incoming EMR documents? How will non-patient documents and faxes (e.g., Medicare EOBs) be stored in the imaging feature of the EMR?
Quality Assurance	What are the daily procedures to insure the maintenance of medical records on a timely basis? What are the documentation requirements for various chief complaints and diseases? How will the practice monitor outstanding issues and completion of overdue items?
Practice Management	What are the performance and operational standards that should be monitored during the working day? How should overdue tasks and orders be handled? How will management evaluate the performance of the practice on a retrospective basis?

By mapping the EMR workflow upfront, you will create a structure and standard for the implementation effort as well as catalogue issues that will be addressed during implementation. Workflow documents allow you to map something you know about (your current clinical processes) with a vision based on your general knowledge of the EMR product. For example, you know the types of outside documents that are received by the practice and added to the paper record. However, such documents are not currently tracked or managed. If those documents could be tracked, what would you want to know about their status, who would be responsible for managing the flow and how would the documents be organized? The answers to these questions would determine a number of setups in any EMR product. The workflow will be refined and detailed as you move forward. The workflow document will facilitate a closer match of the product to your practice.

The workflow document establishes the reference point for your further EMR efforts. The workflow document will affect your hardware setups, software options, training and data conversion strategies. Indeed, the workflow document will ultimately be used to create the detailed written procedures that are your key to compliance with the HIPAA Privacy and Security standards.

FACILITIES MANAGEMENT

EMRs require facility accommodations to protect your investment as well as practically support the EMR.

The first priority should be securing the EMR servers and other key equipment. The typical PMS system is kept any place the practice has room. Practices keep their PMS systems and network servers in employee offices, medical file rooms, hallways, lunch rooms and just about any other place in the practice.

On the regulatory side, the HIPAA Security Standards include physical security guidelines that should be considered for your practice. You should seriously consider how to protect your EMR from an accident that could damage you equipment or allow inappropriate disclosures. In addition to the HIPAA standards, you want to avoid an incident that could disrupt operations and impact patient service. EMR based facility issues include:

Secured Computer Room—Due to the mission critical nature of the EMR, your practice should protect the system from physical and environmental risks. Your computer room should be separated from areas frequented by staff and patients. The room should not include printers and workstations that increase traffic. The computer room should include a solid core door with a lock and be large enough to allow for quick access to the equipment. In some cases, practices squeeze the EMR systems into the small room that currently hosts the PMS. You should seriously consider improvements that mitigate the risk of problems from environmental factors:

Security Alarm—The computer room should be protected with a security alarm system. Depending on office access issues, you may connect the alarm to the general office access controls.

Limited Access—Computer room access should be limited to a few select and trained supervisors and managers. The computer room should not contain any equipment (e.g., printers, scanners, workstations) that would require regular access and use by others.

Fire Protection—Computers can be damaged by water from fire sprinklers. To avoid damage from water, the practice should consider a waterless fire suppression system ($7,000-$10,000).

Air Conditioning—Servers and other computer equipment can generate enough heat to cause equipment problems and automatic shutdown. The computer room may need supplemental air conditioning to compensate for the equipment. Supplemental air conditioning may be supplied by an extra vent or an additional unit. **ALERT:** Adequate air flow is an important consideration for any air conditioning evaluation. You need to insure that the cabinets are not positioned to cause "hot spots" that could damage your equipment.

Direct Circuits—Power outlets should use direct circuits to prevent power disruptions from other equipment on the same circuit. Even with power conditioning equipment such as uninterruptible power supplies, many practices should use a direct circuit to mitigate many variables on a cost effective basis.

Uninterruptible Power Supplies (UPS)—UPSs mitigate the possibility of power disruptions to system operations. Depending on the reliability of power in your facility, you may seek a 15 minute or more power supply. The UPS must be powerful enough to support the complete operation of the system. For example, you may need power for a router and a workstation to access the system as well. *TIP:* UPSs have significant limitations since they cannot reasonably run the air conditioning in the room. For example, buying 4 hours of UPS services will not be very useful if the room will become too hot for the equipment 30 minutes after the power fails. Some practices connect to a UPS backed up by an on demand generator to insure the system is still operational for a long period of time even if the building loses power.

Backup Communications—Remote offices may connect to the EMR over a fast line to service all users. The practice may choose to use a backup communications channel that provides a lower level of service, but supports continued operations. For example, you may suspend scanning during a communications problem with the primary communications line and switch to a slower DSL line. *TIP:* The backup communications line should be through a different service that the line you are backing up. Otherwise, a single point of failure could cut off both lines: you would have paid two for a service with the same risk factors.

Offsite Server Hosting—In some cases, you may move the computer servers to a hosting site that provides the various safeguards that are listed above. Your servers would be hosted at the site for a monthly fee. Note that you may incur additional communication expenses for the high speed line between your office and the host site.

Training Room—Regardless of your setup and training plan, you will need to have an onsite training room for your staff. The room will be used for the initial training as well as teaching of new employees and continuing training needed for your employees. You may choose to set aside a conference room or other location. Bigger practices with several large locations may establish more than one training room. The training room should feature the equipment in use with the EMR. Sufficient workstations and tablet access, as well as scanners and printers, should be available. Note that the training room can also be used as a staging area for the initial entry of information and/or scanning.

Clinical Office—EMR users require appropriate workspace. *TIP*: Account for practical places to put tablets in the exam rooms as well as surfaces to work in the hallways. You should also validate the location of workstations according to workflow and user viewing needs. For example, some practices install a workstation at the clinical working areas even if all staff use tablets. The workstation with a larger screen may be used to view diagnostic images. Don't forget a convenient location for printers to be used by staff as well as adequate locations for workstations. Note that the current locations and shelving used for medical record storage may be useful for the EMR equipment. For example, you may be able to place a printer at a clinical desk that is currently stacked with medical records. Patients may need to see a screen to view patient education aides when the doctor is explaining a condition or procedure.

Front desk—Incoming documents from patients will be scanned at the front desk into the EMR. In many situations, space at the front desk is at a premium. However, each front desk station will require a scanner to capture incoming documents. Note that the entire front desk setup should be reviewed since additional patient service work will be performed there. For example, patients may be providing completed forms that will be scanned into the EMR in support of the office visit. If the front desk can not accommodate scanning, then you may need to perform front desk scanning elsewhere in the office. However, you need to insure that the incoming documents can be scanned before the patient is seen.

Reception Area—The practice should consider installing one or more workstations in the reception area for patients. The workstations could be used by patients to access information on the practice, as well as information on various clinical conditions. For example, online patient education for various procedures could be accessed. Some EMR systems support patient information entry into the EMR. Typically, the patient is given a unique number, and accesses a Web Site to enter information and answer questions. Web-based information entry may allow for changes to demographics, appointment requests, refill requests, communications with doctors and staff, as well as viewing lab results and recall issues. Patient information is held for review by the doctor before acceptance into the EMR. In order to support the entry of information, the practice may need workstations in a private area for patients.

Medical records—If your practice will scan the patient charts into the EMR, the medical records area will need a major redesign. Most medical record areas lack adequate space for scanning. ***CAUTION:*** Depending on your strategy, medical record scanning could be very intense for at least 6 months after EMR Go Live. Medical record scanning requires preparing the chart for scanning, the scanning of the chart, connecting the chart to the patient and preparing the scanned chart for storage or destruction. Considering that a substantial number of charts will be partially or completely scanned daily, you need to insure that sufficient space is available. You will need space to pull charts several days in advance as well as to hold charts that have been prepared for scanning, but need to be scanned. A major problem for many practices is storing the scanned charts and preventing further access after scanning. Unfortunately, you will need to allow for extra space for these functions before shelf space is freed up to support the scanning process. Note that areas and surfaces used to organize charts for refiling and the entire filing process will change with an EMR. ***TIP:*** Some practices use a conference room, or temporarily rent space from another practice to support chart scanning.

Office facilities are part of the infrastructure needed to support you EMR effort. Some of these facilities will be driven by HIPAA standards.

TECHNOLOGY BASE

EMR installation triggers a dramatic expansion and upgrade to the practice technology base. To support an EMR, you will certainly add new servers, workstations and tablets as well as the network and peripherals needed to support clinical workflow. You will also make hardware investments to "harden" your system and insure continued access to the medical records in case of a variety of system problems and/or failures. The following issues should be noted as you work on your technology base:

Server Availability—You should closely examine your server and network setup for the weakest link and review the possibility of a problem. Even if you have invested a substantial amount of money in the EMR server, your entire system could be at risk for the failure due to a relatively inexpensive component. For example, one practice suffered a system crash due to a failure in the Active Directory Server, which could have been prevented by a small investment.

Communications—An EMR will generate much more computer traffic between your sites and the location of the EMR Server(s.) Additional traffic is due to more users, more use of the EMR by each user and the use of images. Communication changes typically have the longest lead times of any of the hardware areas. Changes can take at least 30 days without accounting for the labyrinth of vendors you may have to deal with. Unfortunately, you may lack any quantitative information until the system has been installed. However, a careful review of the vendor's recommendation and monitoring use as the EMR is activated will help you anticipate a problem before your practice is affected. For example, some vendors recommend a certain amount of communication bandwidth for each user at a remote site. You should verify that your communication plan allows for the requisite service. **ALERT:** Some communication services can be quickly upgraded from a remote location, while new services can take up to 90 days to install. Make sure that communication orders are properly placed on the critical path for the EMR project.

Workstations and Tablets—Virtually everyone in the practice will need access to the EMR. Many employees will need access to both EMR and PMS. For example, clinical staff may schedule patients for procedures as well as work with the medical record. Workstations and wireless tablets offer users different access options according to their needs. In general, desktop workstations are appropriate for doctors and staff that primarily work in a specific location. Wireless tablets are useful for doctors and staff who move around the facility. **ALERT:** The appropriateness of the device can be effected by the EMR software. For example, some EMR products are easier to use with a stylus or touchscreen than with a mouse. Selected EMR products are designed to let a nurse record information, and turn over the workstation at the current step in the record to a doctor. When looking at a specific user, the practice needs to exam the user's role. Of course, the user has to be comfortable with his situation. For example, a desktop station in an exam room may be difficult for a user who moves from room-to-room with different patients. In other situations, a mid-level nurse, PA and/or tech may actually document the patient visit as the doctor is working with the patient. This user may be more comfortable with a workstation. Note that maintaining confidentiality for workstations requires users secure the workstation from access by unauthorized users before they leave the exam room. In some cases, you can enforce security standards by automatically shutting down the user after a period of inactivity (e.g., 5 minutes or 30 minutes).

Scanners—The key benefit and objective of an EMR is the paperless office. Even if you succeed in establishing a paperless office, your patients, trading partners and other organizations will continue to send you an avalanche of paper (e.g., ER reports, consulting doctor reports, diagnostic test results) and demand paper from you. Initially, you will need scanner capacity to scan paper medical records as well as scan relevant paper received by your practice. A fax server allows you to receive faxes and load the fax image into the EMR without printing a fax or the need to scan it. However, you will need to have scanners available to capture paper documents and enter the information into the patient record.

The installation of hardware and system software will evolve over the course of the project. Although you can expect few changes to your EMR servers, other items will depend on the EMR workflow and user preferences. For example, most products will print a consent form that is signed by the patient and scanned into the EMR. You would need a scanner that could be conveniently used to scan the consent form or a computer signing pad to record signed consents. The key factors affecting the technology include the lead time for items, final hardware decisions and the general implementation plan for the practice. If you are using more than one vendor for hardware, the technology effort will be more complex, since you will have to coordinate the two or more vendors and insure that all of the purchased products work together. ***TIP:*** Make sure that orders from multiple vendors are properly coordinated by an appropriate IT coordinator to insure that the products are correctly installed.

During the contracting process, the EMR vendor supplied hardware specifications for its system. If hardware is being purchased from another source, you should have verified the items purchased with the EMR vendor. As you proceed to finalize your technology base, you should consider the issues listed in Table 9.6.

Installation of the hardware is a complex affair due to the number of changes and EMR setup issues. For example, some EMRs have a special piece of software that must be installed in each workstation and tablet. If you are buying all equipment from the EMR vendor, then you don't have too much to worry about. If you are buying the components from multiple vendors, then you need to plan the sequence of the installation to insure that you do not cause work stoppages or penalties from other vendors. The hardware installation plan should account for the following:

1. The primary network, workstation and tablet vendor should install enough hardware to test connectivity with the EMR Server before the EMR Server is in-

TABLE 9.6

Area	TECHNOLOGY ISSUES TO CONSIDER
Policies	Does the practice have a policy on upgrades and changes to the technology base? What is the technology replacement strategy, and policy for the practice? What is the strategy for accessing the EMR? What hardware components are needed to support the policy? What are the lines of responsibility for the installation and support of the EMR hardware?
Servers	What additional servers are needed for the EMR besides the equipment being purchased from the EMR vendor? Are current network servers (e.g., active directory server, print and file server, email server) adequate for the EMR and the anticipated larger user-base? Do the number of users warrant additional facilities for remote users, communications, printing services, and availability of workstations/tablets? If using a communications server (e.g., Windows Terminal Server or Citrix), which workstations and tablets will work through the communications server to the EMR? Does the backup device capacity and strategy account for all of the servers on the practice network? What is the strategy to protect the servers and workstations from virus, spyware and other intrusive software?
PMS	Does the PMS system require an upgrade before the EMR is installed? What, if any, equipment is needed to support the EMR interface? What is the working relationship between the PMS and EMR systems and vendors? Do the code sets and master files used by the PMS require changes before the PMS is interfaced with the EMR? Do the triggers for sending data between the EMR and PMS systems adequately support the use of both systems for patients in the office?
Communications	Are the communication links between offices sufficient for the EMR? Are adequate protections in place to prevent intrusion or disruptions from outside sources? Is there adequate network protection through firewalls and internal security? Do the internal network facilities in each location have the capacity to support an EMR? What are the security features of the network to protect against unauthorized access? What are the wireless network issues in each location? Is there any existing equipment that may interfere with the wireless network?
Workstations	What, if any, upgrades are required to meet the minimum EMR standards? What additional workstations are needed to support the EMR? What screens will provide the best view of EMR data and images? What other initiatives (Ex. PACS, new diagnostic equipment, access to hospital information) could affect the number and placement of workstations?
Tablets	What criterion determines tablet use by a user? What is the deployment plan for tablet distribution? How will doctors and staff who work in multiple locations use tablets? What is needed to provide adequate wireless access to the users in the office and related areas (e.g., lunch room)?
Scanners	Where will scanners be needed to scan incoming documents into the EMR? What scanning devices will be needed in medical records for old paper charts? What is the planned scanning throughput that will be available for medical record scanning? How will the scanners fit in the medical records department and other areas?
Printers	Where will patient materials be printed? What printers will be needed to support EMR printing requirements?

stalled on your network. The primary hardware vendor should allow for a resource to work with the EMR vendor when the EMR Server is installed.

2. Insure that your internal technical support person works with the EMR vendor on the installation of the EMR Server. Your internal technical support person should understand the general setup of the EMR server and the requirements for the various devices that access the EMR. **TIP:** Most practices need a higher level support person on call to address any issues that cannot be resolved by the internal resource.

3. The internal technical support person and your primary hardware vendor should understand the various tasks needed to stage, prepare and configure a device to access or use the EMR.

The final proof of the hardware setup is when the entire system is hooked together. When the EMR Server(s) and infrastructure are available for use, your practice should verify the delivery and operability of the EMR system using your own staff as shown in Table 9.7.

TABLE 9.7

Area	VERIFYING TECHNOLOGY INSTALLATION
General	All equipment should be verified against the list of equipment ordered from each vendor. Verify that: • Each server, workstation and tablet contains the ordered memory, disks, and other features. • Each scanner and printer is the ordered model and/or meets the order specifications. • Interfaces with diagnostic equipment are properly connected and working. • Servers can be backed up with the back-up equipment and the backup is valid.
Servers	Verify the ordered equipment and operability of high availability options, such as dual power supplies, dual fans and hot swap disk arrays. Verify that all servers are communicating with the network at the expected speed. Verify that all servers can access other servers as needed (e.g., PMS and EMR servers). Verify that the PMS and EMR systems exchange information on a timely basis through the purchased interface.
PMS	Insure that the appropriate EMR workstations can still access the PMS system as needed. Verify the interface between the PMS and EMR system for appointments, demographics and charges.
Communications	Verify interoffice communication links operate at the expected speeds. Verify network speeds in offices support use of the EMR.
Workstations	Check that upgraded workstations can operate with the EMR. Verify that the EMR and PMS products can be run simultaneously on workstations that will require simultaneous access to both applications. Test printing to appropriate printers for each workstation. Verify viewing of EMR information and images.
Tablets	Verify wireless access and operation of the EMR on each tablet. Test printing to appropriate printers for each tablet.
Scanners	Test the ability to scan a document into the EMR. Verify the quality of scanning and the stored image in the EMR meet the clarity and precision needs of the practice.
Printers	Verify printing reports from the EMR to selected printers. Check the default printer for the user as well as the availability of appropriate network printing resources.

After confirmation of the hardware installation, written documentation on installation of equipment and maintenance issues should be developed for the EMR. The documentation should include instructions on the hardware requirements, software installation and connectivity setups. Make sure you also compile information on system backup and recovery. You should also compile a list of key contact numbers, vendors and names to help staff in the event of a system problem.

SOFTWARE SETUP

Software setup involves selecting from a variety of EMR options and classification tools to customize the EMR for your practice. Although system features and setup options vary, several options are available on most EMR products:

Security—The security setup can be derived from the workflow document. The workflow document lays out what each person in each area will be doing. The workflow document can be used to define roles, which are included in the security setup. Some EMRs allow restrictions based on record types, locations, patient types and doctors. Security restrictions at these levels should be based on practice policies and the recommendation of your security officer. **TIP:** The practice should have a formal document that defines access rights for each type of employee as well as a formal process to give selected employees specific rights or additional capabilities.

Imaging—Imaging modules support scanned images from paper records, incoming documents and diagnostic images. To keep track of the various images, you can define image types. To organize image types, you should compile a list of the types of images that you want to be able to select immediately from the patient EMR chart (e.g., office notes by date, diagnostic reports by problem). At a minimum, you need image types for the old medical record (e.g., old office notes, old lab results), incoming reports, letters from physicians (such as referral letters) and letters from patients. You may also define image types for audiograms, patient information sheets, radiology reports and ER documents. To compile a report list, scan through your paper medical record and note the types of documents that you would want to be able to immediately access. You may also have non-clinical documents among the EMR images. For example, a referral authorization from an insurer or a scanned image of the insurance card may be stored in an EMR. Some imaging products allow for a free form description. The practice should establish a standard format for the description (e.g., "Shoulder X-ray—Central Radiology"). Other imaging modules allow you to define a specific set of data items for each image type. For example, you could enter the hospital name and date of service for an ER report and the optical lab and due date for a custom optical product.

Tasks—Tasks record "to do" items in an EMR. Tasks may be assigned to one or more people and labeled according to a priority. These classify tasks to allow the recipient to immediately identify the nature of the task as well as allow management to print reports by task type. Task types may address incoming documents (e.g., "Review a Lab Report"), clinical communications ("Approve a Mid-Level Note"), patient service ("Refill Request") and patient treatment ("Perform Lab Test," "Schedule Surgery Request," "Waiting for an X-Ray," etc.). Make sure that the list addresses ancillary services, and the vast array of interactions on patient issues. The list should be organized into groups to keep the number of task types to a manageable number. **ALERT:** Some products have multiple options to flag tasks that are needed by larger practices. For example, you may be able to assign a priority, department, and type to a task. If a product only allows for a short description line, then a larger practice may have difficulty tracking patients.

Department Areas and Locations—EMR setup should reflect your department and location setup. However, you should consider the operational departments that would facilitate use of the EMR. For example, you may have a diagnostic pod that contains lab, radiology and ultrasound, but in your operational analysis, you may be better off making them separate EMR departments. **TIP:** The use of departments may not be fully developed in the EMR. For example, if you can assign departments, but cannot view patients and tasks by department, then department will not be as useful. If you can view patients, tasks, documents, and other items by department, the EMR will support more effective management tools for the practice.

Appointment Tracking—Some EMRs include patient flow features within the EMR appointment scheduler. You may be able to enter a patient status, room number and/or comment. Complile a list of meaningful statuses that reflects the possible situations a patient may encounter in your facility (e.g., "Roomed," "Technician Intake," "Waiting for Doctor," "Procedure Pending." etc.). Use statuses that apply across several departments. For example, a general status of waiting for a test that could apply to the lab and radiology is preferable to a separate "waiting for test" status for each department. The department should be communicated through the assigned area and/or room assignment. **ALERT:** You may want to consider how you identify and classify the various departments of your practice. For example, if each room in each office is separately listed in the EMR, then you may be faced with a long list of rooms when you want to record a patient move in the EMR. However, if the EMR tracks the location and pod of the patient, you may be able to use a shorter list of room numbers that are standardized across all practice locations.

Plan Items—When a doctor is recording a plan for a patient, she may select procedures, tests, patient education, recall appointments and other actions to support patient care. These plan items should be compiled from existing records to speed the EMR setup process. Plan items may include lab tests, radiology studies and treatments. Plan items lists may be assigned to diseases and/or physicians depending on the EMR. The plan items should be standardized across all doctors to ease management of patient care. For example, support staff needs to be able to easily identify pending treatment items without having to deal with different coding systems for the same plan item. Note that plan items should relate to or be associated with the evolving care standards that may be used in your area. You will be better positioned to track and manage the evolving quality of care and pay-for-performance initiatives.

Software interfaces will require appropriate setups and testing. Setup may include programming the various interfaces as well as compiling translation tables to support interfaces. The interfaces should be mostly managed by the EMR, PMS and diagnostic equipment vendors. The EMR project manager will be mostly responsible for coordinating the various parties on the following interfaces:

PMS Interface—The PMS system should send patient demographic and appointment information to the EMR. The EMR should send charge information to the PMS. The software interface should work fast enough to allow a patient at check-in to be properly reflected in the EMR system as well as transfer a charge from the EMR to the PMS in time for patient checkout.

Diagnostic Equipment Interfaces—Diagnostic equipment interfaces with the EMR should allow downloading of the results to the EMR or viewing the diagnostic results from the EMR in time to support review by the doctor. Note that many EMRs do not necessarily save the diagnostic image, but store a pointer to the diagnostic image on the diagnostic equipment. When you select the diagnostic image from the EMR, the EMR invokes the diagnostic image viewer and the user is now viewing the patient image through the diagnostic equipment tools. ***ALERT:*** Such connections mean that the results on the diagnostic equipment are de facto extensions of the EMR. However, you need to adequately backup the images on the diagnostic equipment to maintain the integrity of the patient's medical record. In some cases, your EMR can send the order information with the patient identification to the diagnostic equipment to eliminate duplicate information entry. ***TIP:*** Insure that you purchase diagnostic equipment interfaces with your EMR and future purchases of diagnostic equipment should include the interface needed for the EMR.

The clinical content should be carefully reviewed to avoid problems during the training and deployment effort. Clinical content review and acceptance requires active involvement of doctors and clinical staff. The medical staff dedicated to the EMR implementation effort should lead the following effort:

Review the Current Clinical Content—Super user doctors and other clinical staff should review the EMR clinical content for their designated area. The clinical content review should cover the applicability of the clinical content to the practice as well as nuances that may be required. For example, a patient population that is at a high risk for a particular disease may require some additional information in the EMR. Similarly, a subspecialist needs to review the content in the EMR for his area. As the review is conducted, the user should take notes on enhancements and changes needed to meet practice requirements. Enhancements should be noted between those items that are a necessity and those items that would be useful, but are not needed immediately. For example, the resulting note may not be exactly how the doctor would have transcribed the issue, but may correctly reflect the patient's situation. **CAUTION:** Many practices start off customizing the clinical content without fully understanding the "out of the box" clinical content. You could end up customizing the clinical content for something that already exists. Before you invest time and resources in any custom content, make sure you understand what the purchased system does and evaluate whether it would work for you. **TIP:** Note that the clinical content may work, but may be different from how you would do it yourself. If the clinical content accurately documents the patient condition and treatment, you may save a lot of time and effort accepting the standard, instead of customizing the EMR content to reflect how you would have designed or set up the EMR.

Design Changes—If changes and enhancements are needed, describe the list of enhancements in as much detail as possible to avoid problems and mistakes. For example, you may request that a flag for diabetes be added between the heart problem and arthritis questions instead of stating that "diabetes is not included on the problem list."

Implement Changes or Setups—The vendor and/or trained practice staff will program the changes into the EMR clinical content. Be careful to monitor the effect that multiple requests may have on a screen or clinical content list to avoid redoing work. For example, some practices rework areas several times (at additional cost) before arriving at a workable solution. The implementation of the change should have a specific delivery date, and you should have a specific test to verify the change. For example, you may include an example of what the resulting screen and document will look like. **TIP:** Most practices will need an internal resource that understands how to customize and enhance the clinical content. However, those changes should be carefully designed and evaluated by the clinical users, before the practice invests time in changes that may already be available in the EMR, or may not add much to EMR utility. For example, a user may want to see a particular piece of information in a certain place in a selected screen even though the information can be viewed on another screen within the EMR.

Test Changes—After setting up the various clinical content system options or customizations, the doctors should test the EMR to validate the handling of clinical issues. The testing will allow the physician to verify the content, and gain confidence in the EMR. The testing should include a variety of key clinical areas. Several testing strategies should be considered:

Retrospective Records—Previously documented encounters will be entered into the EMR to verify the ability to document a visit. The resulting report will be reviewed by the doctor to analyze the result in light of the actual chart note. Know that the new system will not necessarily produce the exact note, but an accurate and correct document.

Role Playing—A medical exam will be conducted in a conference room setting with a doctor or clinician recording the information being presented by another practice clinician. The purpose of role playing is to test the flow of the EMR in an interactive environment with the ability to backtrack and rework the "exam" with the EMR.

Patient Shadowing—An actual patient visit is shadowed with the EMR. The user will record the patient information in the EMR at the same time other records are kept by the doctor performing the services. The resulting record is reviewed to verify that the note and record are acceptable to the practice.

Document Production—If the clinical charting is working well in testing, the practice may try documenting patient visits using the EMR. The EMR will be used to produce the report that will be saved in the paper chart until the practice moves to the EMR. This strategy maintains the integrity of the designated record set.

EMR software setup is particularly sensitive due to the importance of the clinical content. The effort involved in verifying and testing the clinical content with the practice's clinical information and treatment strategies will mitigate the chance of a failure as the practice moves forward with the activation of the EMR.

DATA CONVERSION

EMR Data conversion is more complicated that anything that you may have encountered with a practice management system (PMS). The implementation of a new PMS system involves the manual or electronic conversion of information from the old PMS to the new PMS. The old PMS has a patient demographic record and so does the new PMS. Indeed, the new PMS data structures and items are generally analogous to the old PMS.

Current medical record information primarily consists of paper patient charts. Some practices may also have electronic patient information in a number of places. For example, you may have transcription files, test results in lab information systems and various images in selected diagnostic testing devices. Converting to an EMR will be difficult and complex. You need to carefully review the options and understand what you will have at the end of the effort.

Initially, the practice should determine what information you need to move to the EMR and where the information is currently stored. As a practical matter, the current information could consist of the following:

Paper Record Conversion—Conversion of paper records is covered in a separate section below.

Transcription Files—Some practices have transcripted word processing files that may go back several years. Ideally, these records should be a valuable basis of information that could be loaded as a starting point into the EMR. However, many practices have procedures that could undermine the utility of these saved files.

> **Editing and Side Notes**—If the electronic document could differ in any way from the patient chart document, the conversion of the electronic document could cause inconsistencies in the EMR and expose the practice to problems. Practices where the doctor may edit the final chart document by hand, or note additional information on the chart document should be wary of any electronic conversion. Similarly, doctors who record supplemental notes, phone calls and other information on the bottom of the transcribed note may not be able to rely on the electronic version of the note as the most current patient information.

> **Certainty of the Document**—Word processing documents are not secured from access or change in the vast majority of practices. Indeed, small changes could be introduced in a variety of scenarios that created differences between the electronic document and the document in the patient chart. For example, some practices maintain a single file for a patient and append new dictation to the end of the document. However, there is no mechanism to prevent changes to information that is already in the word processing file.

> **Document Organization**—Some practices use a single file to store all doctor dictation in a day or on a tape. If the separation between patients is not clearly indicated and consistent, the separation of the documents may be complicated or produce inconsistent results. Indeed, some vendors cannot support electronic conversion of transcription files unless a file only contains a single document for a single date of service for an easily identified patient.

> **Patient Identification**—To support computerized loading of transcription files into an EMR, patient identification must be clear and certain. Patient name alone will not be sufficient. The patient name, medical record number, sex and date of birth in a consistent place will enable the electronic loading of the word processing files into the EMR. Most practices do not include a complete complement of patient information in each transcribed document.

In the final analysis, any differences between the saved transcription files and the patient paper chart could lead to problems. If your practice does not save transcription files that could be electronically converted, you should consider changing procedures to insure the reliability and accuracy of future electronic documents. You may be able to electronically convert the transcription files from the point of the changes with confidence in the reliability of the document.

Lab Information System (LIS)—Practice-owned LISs contain lab results that predate the EMR. If previous results could be loaded into the EMR, then doctors could use the graphing tools to review trends, as well as look at previous lab results in the lab flow-sheets. With an interface that links LIS results to your EMR, the old results from the LIS could be downloaded into the EMR. The loading would add a considerable amount of patient information as well as test the LIS interface. However, the EMR must be able to accept lab results for tests that were not ordered through the EMR.

Diagnostic Equipment—Some diagnostic equipment store information and images from previous tests. Diagnostic equipment in the typical practice may support an electronic interface with an EMR, or support a workaround strategy that creates an image file that can be loaded into an EMR. In some cases, the diagnostic equipment cannot support any interface. Diagnostic equipment with interfaces to the EMR could be used to download previous results into the EMR. Otherwise, the previous results must be printed or exported to a computer file for transfer to the new EMR.

Master Files—In many cases, EMR master files must be manually established and maintained. EMR Master Files may include procedures, diagnoses, doctors, locations and insurance companies. Some EMR vendors may load selected PMS Master File information, such as insurance company, diagnoses and procedures, into the EMR at installation. Note that even when PMS systems update the EMR master files, the scheduling may cause problems. For example, some vendors update the records on a daily or even a weekly basis. If the additional information is needed sooner, the EMR may just ignore the unknown master file code. For example, a new payer added to the master file would not connect the patient with the correct medication formulary if the payer and formulary in the EMR is not updated on a continual basis.

Demographic Information—Some EMRs have an independent demographic information database that can be maintained through the EMR. A limited number of products rely exclusively on the PMS interface for demographic information. With an interfaced EMR, all current PMS patient information must be loaded into the EMR. Otherwise, patients who have not been seen since the EMR's implementation will not be accessible through the EMR. Phone messages, incoming results and other information could not be entered into the EMR prior to the patient's first post-EMR Go Live visit. Note that integrated PMS and EMR products share the same demographic and master files. Information entered in either area is immediately accessible to the other EMR components. ***ALERT:*** Most EMR interfaces do not send demographic updates to the EMR. However, EMR users may update EMR demographic information but not remember that the updates will not be passed to the PMS. This problem is especially troublesome when EMR users frequently access the EMR demographics and may even add information to the EMR demographics as part of using the EMR. For example, you may go into the EMR to maintain an alert message or add information that is not even contained in the PMS (Ex. Preferred pharmacy.) While updating the EMR demographic information, the user could accidentally update some information (Ex. Address or contact phone) that should be posted to the PMS. Another related problem can be exposed when the triage staff answers a patient call and gets a new phone number for the patient. The new number has to be associated with the patient message in the EMR, but the new number has to be separately posted to the PMS.

Appointment Information—With an interfaced EMR, the current appointments should be sent to the EMR. After the initial appointments, changes to the appointment schedule will trigger the maintenance of the EMR appointments for each PMS appointment change. The appointment schedule enables patient workflow management through the EMR. Note that the key issue for any interface is the trigger mechanism. In some cases, changes to some appointment information may not necessarily trigger an update to the EMR appointment schedule. For example, an update to the appointment time will certainly trigger an update to the EMR, but the entry of a note may not be sent to the EMR from the PMS. *TIP:* In most cases, PMS systems do not track patient progress through the office and at the most only know that the patient has presented for service. PMS products that support check-in will send the check-in information to the EMR. However, PMS systems that do not support patient check-in are more challenging. If the PMS does not support check-in, then the front desk staff will have to access the appointment information in the EMR to check the patient in. The EMR check-in status indicates to the clinical staff that the patient is ready to be seen.

Depending on the ability to convert this information, you could start off with some significant EMR patient data on EMR Go Live. However, the practice needs to plan ahead to enable the conversion of data into the EMR.

PAPER CHARTS AND THE EMR

EMR structures and data collection strategies are completely different from the current paper-based methods. For example, many EMRs maintain separate lists of medications, diagnoses, procedures, allergies and other key patient information. This information is typically buried in various places in the paper record. Even practices that maintain separate logs of medications and key patient information (Ex. Immunization, Previous Surgery) cannot be absolutely sure that the paper chart contains information that has not been entered in the logs. Indeed, some practices have procedures to check the records to make the logs are complete before the patient is seen. The maintenance of such logs is often inconsistent and prone to errors. For example, an obsolete medications' log may present a misleading view of the patient situation and risks, if staff fails to update the log after the last visit. In many cases, you cannot even tell the last time such logs were checked or verified.

Converting paper medical charts requires a complex and time consuming effort. The key issue to consider is what information you need from the current paper charts, and what effort will be invested to get the information into the EMR. Information from paper charts are entered into the EMR as a scanned image of the paper records, and/or as discrete information from the paper records (e.g., medications). For example, a practice may decide to scan the medical chart into the EMR, but also review the EMR to enter the patient's medical history into the chart. In some cases, the practice will not really have a choice about entering specific information into the EMR. For example, a pediatric practice must enter the patient immunization information into the EMR. Otherwise, the health maintenance rules may flag patients who "need" immunization shots as far as the EMR knows, but could be up to date according to the patient paper record.

Virtually no practice sets up their paper records to facilitate or support scanning. For example, paper charts lack consistent patient identifiers on the individual chart pages. The organization of the paper chart may complicate scanning. For example, practices may keep paper records in the order received and not by visit, condition or type of document. In some cases, practices maintain family charts where patient information is commingled with information from other family members. Other practices may maintain "case" charts for each patient problem. As a practical matter, a number of practices maintain separate charts in each office for each patient seen in each office. If a patient is seen in more than one office, they could end up with more than one chart. The paper medical record poses a number of challenges to scanning including:

A variety of paper sizes—Paper size differences can slow the scanning process or leave awkward images. For example, a limited number of legal-sized pages may have to be separately scanned from the rest of the chart or regular-sized images may appear to have empty space at the bottom of each page. Undersized prescriptions, tapes from diagnostic equipment and other undersized documents may have to be taped to a more scanner friendly form.

Two-sided images—Some charts contain information on both sides of some pages. To scan information on both sides of the page the staff may copy the second side, or use a dual-sided scanner to scan both sides of a page in one pass. However, with dual scanning, blank second sides may also end up in the scanned record. Some scanners include software that will identify blank pages according to a specific standard or tolerance. In other cases, a "blank" second side may be a form that does not contain information but will not be considered empty by the scanning software. An additional complication may occur when the second side is upside down to simplify review of paper charts. In the scanned image, the second page will be scanned upside down with dual-sided scanning. An EMR user will have to rotate the image to see the image right side up.

Unnecessary Information—Many practices have charts with duplicate information and obsolete data that has never been removed. For example, the chart may contain patient information and insurance cards from years ago, or various reports that were superseded by interim or final reports. In some cases, practices make copies of medical chart contents for Release of Information and return copies of all information sent in the paper chart. Other charts contain copies of chart pages that were scanned or faxed to other offices and returned to the paper chart. The additional images may complicate locating the information needed in much the same way that the doctor has to leaf through the extraneous documents in a paper chart.

Information on the file folder—Many practices record key patient information on the front, back and/or inside covers of the medical chart. Key medical issues, procedure history, allergies and prescription stickers are some of the items placed on medical chart folders. Unfortunately, the chart folder is difficult to scan. The chart must be placed on a flat-bed scanner and scanned a surface at a time.

Loose documents/forms—Some paper charts contain loose pages that are in the middle of the chart. The appropriate place for the loose pages is not always certain. In other cases, the patient chart is a collection of unsecured pages. The practice may have a clinical staff person "prepare" the chart for each visit by reorganizing some of the loose pages into an order the doctor prefers. Note that the staff may be continually reorganizing the chart for each patient visit and as new information is collected in the chart.

Curled papers—Over time, chart papers can curl, bend or become worn. Such pages will require more time to prepare for scanning since the paper feed is sensitive to paper quality. Ultimately, more paper feeding problems may be encountered as the documents are scanned.

Stapled documents—Staples and paper clips must be removed from documents when scanning. You may be able to save some prep time by tearing off the stapled corner of a document instead of removing a staple.

Poor copies—Paper medical records commonly include poor or aged documents that are difficult to read. Examples include faxed images of EKGs, copies of documents in poor condition, and old thermal paper images. Carbon pages may be of poor quality and difficult to read. Such documents may not scan well.

Color images—Color images in a paper file need to be scanned using a color scanning option. Depending on the placement of images and scanning strategy, all images may be scanned using a color option. Although more convenient, scanning in color generates much larger files even when the document may not contain any color. For example, a black and white scanned image may take up as little as 10,000 characters for a page. However, a color image could consume 1,000 times as much space or even more.

Dividers—Dividers may help or hurt the scanning process depending on your scanning and organization strategy. If you decide to split out more recent records from older clinical information, dividers may increase prep time. If you plan to scan images into sections that are the same as your dividers, then the dividers will speed the scanning process.

Slides—Slides that are contained in the paper chart can be scanned into the EMR using a special scanning device. But slides and other diagnostic images may add additional steps and time to your scanning effort.

Initially, the chart contents must be prepared for scanning. Depending on the chart order and the scanning strategy, the preparation effort can vary widely. At a minimum, you have to remove staples and paperclips as well as straighten the papers to feed the scanner. Other preparation strategies may be determined by the equipment you buy, and your scanning strategy. For example,

- One-sided scanners may require copying the back page of patient records to prepare the chart for scanning.
- Paper charts that are not kept in any specific order may require organizing the chart before scanning.
- Paper charts with significant amounts of useless materials may be edited before scanning.
- Some practices used family charts that mix patient information. Such information would have to be separated by patient before scanning.

Whatever your situation or problems, make sure you survey the paper charts to uncover the issues that you will have to deal with and test various paper handling and scanning strategies to determine the best one for you practice. Preparing the paper chart for scanning can easily exceed the time it takes to scan the document. Chart preparation can average 5–30 minutes per chart, depending on the size of the document, and your prep time. Large "phone book" charts could take an hour or more to prepare for scanning.

TIP: Make sure your strategy balances the effort to scan and process the paper record with the resulting benefits of the scanned medical record. ***ALERT:*** Scanning a chart will not make the paper record look better or resolve the paper chart problems of the last 10 years. The resulting scanned images may be kept in a single group of the entire contents of the paper chart or split into various categories. For example, you may choose to have images organized by visit date or by type of document (e.g., office visit, radiology study, lab results, etc.)

Scanners and the target scanner software impact whether you can organize the patient chart before or after you scan the chart into the EMR. Some EMR scanning products only allow you to scan a one page document, while other products allow you to scan an entire chart and use the imaging software to organize the chart. In some cases, scanning software will help you organize the scanned images into groups of images that can be saved in separate folders. For example, you could pick out office notes from the past two years. The recent office notes could be put in one image folder and the rest of the paper chart could be stored in another image folder.

If you cannot organize the scanned images using the scanning software, then you may have to separate a single chart into several individual documents that must be separately scanned into the EMR. In general, scanning individual stacks into separate image folders is more time consuming than scanning the entire chart and using the scanning software to organize the various scanned image folders. Some scanning products use bar coded separator pages to allow you to scan stacks of paper at a time. Without the separators, you may have to use several scanning jobs to separate a single chart into the EMR pieces. These separate jobs will take more scanning time.

Some practices abstract information from the paper record in addition to or as a replacement for scanning. Key information—such as prior medical history, previous procedures, allergies, diagnoses—is entered into the EMR prior to the patient's first visit. In some cases, pulling information from the paper chart is difficult since many documents may be reviewed to gather information. **ALERT:** Entering information from the chart into the EMR will require a clinically experienced person to find the necessary information in the paper chart and follow-up on omissions in the paper chart. The information maybe entered as a dummy prior visit or as the start of the next patient visit. Practices that abstract without scanning frequently maintain a procedure to provide the paper chart on demand to the doctor. If the paper chart is not scanned, you must maintain a paper chart delivery process to insure that doctors can access pre-EMR information for continuity of care issues.

Indeed, some practices do not scan or abstract existing paper records. They merely start using the EMR. The paper records become obsolete for operational purposes, but the practice still keeps the paper chart according to medical record retention laws. The practice is also obligated to maintain the designated record set under the HIPAA privacy standards. In reality, the doctor may still need to go back to the paper chart to review continuity of care issues or a previous problem.

Given all of these issues and difficulties, the average practice would be scared away from doing anything with the current paper records. However, the practice must balance the desire to eliminate paper with the current condition of the paper medical record, and the effort involved with scanning the document. In the final analysis, your scanning strategy or lack thereof will depend on the utility of the final product and the value in the paper record balanced off with the costs of continuing to maintain the paper record after EMR activation. The general scanning options are reviewed in Table 9.8.

In the final analysis, there are no good solutions to the challenge of scanning paper charts into the EMR. If you don't scan anything, you will have to return to the paper chart whenever the doctor needs to research patient issues. If you selectively scan information, you may have to return to the same chart to scan incrementally additional information. If you scan everything, expect the process to take 6–12 months.

Any analysis of your scanning strategy will have to consider the cost of scanning. Using an outside resource, scanned records cost .10 to .30 per image. Depending on the size of your charts the costs could significantly vary for each practice. However, your need to balance the cost of scanning with your continued maintenance and delivery costs for

TABLE 9.8

Option	Strengths	Limitations
No Scanning – Paper records are delivered until they are no longer needed.	No scanning requirements.	• Difficult to manage paper record and tablet. • Information could be written in the paper chart and not into the EMR. For example, a doctor may enter a note in the paper chart to highlight a trend or analyze a result. • Paper charts will never disappear since the paper chart will always be a part of the designated record set. • Managing the designated record set split among the EMR and paper record could be complicated. For example, paper chart information could be used in an encounter documented in the EMR. However, information used in medical decision-making from the paper record would not be in the EMR.
Abstract Paper Records – Important information is entered into the EMR, but the paper record is maintained and delivered to the physician until the paper chart is no longer needed.	Cuts down on accessing the paper chart.	• Consumes doctor or clinician time to prepare the patient record for the first visit. • Information could be missed when abstracted. • Doctor and clinicians would need to see the paper chart for selected patients. For example, the paper chart would contain important trend information for patients with a continuing problem. • Probably requires demand chart delivery in a stat mode for a long period of time. Even after the doctors generally decide the paper charts are no longer needed, the charts will be required on a demand basis. • Any time paper charts are delivered to the doctor or clinician, the practice runs the risk that new information will be recorded in the paper chart. • Difficult maintaining designated record set for each patient since information for EMR based decision-making will be in the patient chart. Paper charts will never disappear since the paper chart will always be a part of the designated record set.
Scan Selected/ Current Information – Based on specific criteria, selected pages are scanned into the EMR. Criteria could include last visit information, all information after a certain date or all office notes. Each time the patient is seen, the doctor could request scanning of additional items from the paper chart.	Fewer EMR images to leaf through when the doctor is scanning the patient chart. Minimizes scanning of information.	• Longer time to select information, scan pages and rebuild the chart. One of the most difficult parts of scanning a paper chart is the preparation of the scanned images. Scanning selected information requires analyzing each document to select the items to be scanned. The selection process could be difficult and open to errors. Putting the chart back together in the order found could be time consuming. • Contextual issues may not be properly reflected in the EMR. Since selected items are scanned, the paper chart may include additional information, interim information or other results that may be needed to fully understand the scanned documents. • Information may not be scanned and could be missed by the doctor looking at only the EMR. • Physicians and medical record staff may need to constantly revisit previously processed charts to scan additional images for a problem already documented in the EMR or to get relevant paper chart information on a problem that is new to the EMR. • Difficult to maintain designated record set. • Paper charts will never disappear.
Limited Medical Record Scanning – Scan some medical records and not others based on some criteria (e.g., size).		• Requires electronic and paper medical record structures and costs. • Any time paper charts are delivered to the doctor or clinician, the practice runs the risk that new information will be recorded in the paper chart. • Requires maintaining paper medical records indefinitely.

Option	Strengths	Limitations
	Patients with smaller charts are scanned into the system, while larger charts can still be reviewed by flipping through the pages of the chart. Alternatively, the practice could establish a selection criteria for patients that trigger the scanning of the entire chart for patients that fit a problem or demographic profile.	• Requires maintaining paper medical records indefinitely. • Difficult to maintain designated record set for patients without scanned charts.
Scan Entire Record – The entire paper medical record is scanned into the EMR based on triggers to insure that the paper record is available when the doctors, clinicians or staff need access to the patient medical record. Note that charts could be scanned using different strategies. For example, a small-to-medium chart could be scanned as a single set of images, while large charts could be separately scanned by section, or current documents could be put in a special section of images.	Maintains designated record set. Once scanned, the paper chart will not have to be accessed again.	• Massive effort needed to scan the records into the EMR. • A variety of problems with scanning productivity since the paper records were not designed for scanning. • Large paper records could be organized into sections at an additional cost and effort.

the paper record. If you expect to pull your charts more than 3 times after you switch over to the EMR, you should closely compare the true cost of pulling, handling, and returning the paper chart with the cost of scanning that same chart.

A number of strategies are available to ease the scanning and record abstraction burden on your practice. Your specific options will depend on your EMR activation strategy (see Chapter 10—Activating an EMR).

TRAINING

EMR training strategies will be impacted by the contract and how you intend to support and train your users. In most practices, a designated group of EMR pioneers is established to champion the EMR implementation effort. These pioneers may be known as key users, super users, champions or a similar term.

Typically, the super users are trained by the vendor. The super users are responsible for setting up the EMR for use, and training the rest of the practice staff. This strategy is quite demanding since the super users must make key decisions on system setup and use as well as train others before they are fully familiar with the EMR.

In some cases, the vendor trains everyone. Most vendor training programs cover all staff on all aspects of the EMR. However, not all users may need to know how to manage and use all EMR features. Training all staff on all features does not let staff concentrate on the specific capabilities that they need to know. Indeed, you may end up training staff on certain capabilities that you may not even want them to know about. For example, setting up security and user access should be limited to a select group of users.

Your EMR training plan should address a number of distinct requirements:

General computer training—Frequently, practice doctors and employees lack the computer skills to use an EMR. Employees may not be comfortable with navigating around the system, using the Windows environment or operating a mouse. You can save money by providing general computer training from a local community college or a training service. Don't use EMR vendors to train your staff on general computer operations. Team staff familiar with the new systems with staff that do not have good computer skills. General computer training will help your staff feel more confident about exploring and using the EMR.

Device Training—Even users who may comfortable using a Windows environment may have problems with some of the new devices that you will be using. For instance, use of a tablet stylus in place of a mouse could pose some issues for various staff members. The best strategy is to give staff time using the various devices. On tablet devices, the user needs to know how to use the stylus, as well as how to change batteries and maintain contact through the wireless network. Other users may need to know how to operate a scanner or work new printers. Device training is best provided by practice staff. Device computer training may help you avoid problems, from connections between devices to turning on and off a device.

Setup Training—Setup training focuses on maintenance of security files, code tables, formularies and charges, as well as system administration. System setup also includes customizing EMR templates, screens, user preferences and practice standards. For example, your practice may design a custom screen to track a certain service that you provide. Setup training is provided by EMR vendors. However, you should limit setup training to a designated group of super users.

In most cases, setup options should be driven by the EMR implementation team and management. EMR setup changes should not be made without the approval of your EMR implementation team. For example, the practice would not want a user to change a set of drug preferences unless the doctors had changed their list. Similarly, an EMR template should not be changed unless the doctors have agreed to the change in clinical documentation and have approved the cost of the change as well as identified tangible benefits from the change.

Application Training—Application training covers using the EMR features and functions. Note that vendor application training will not necessarily address your specific customizations, your workflow strategies or your setup standards. For example, the vendor trainer would cover how to access a clinical template, but the trainer may not understand the clinical details of your template or setups. *TIP:* Make sure your trainer understands the EMR features that will be relevant to your practice and services. For example, a trainer that does not have experience with orthopaedic practices may not have an effective strategy for managing the exchange of patients among orthopedic techs, PAs, and PT staff. Vendors do not typically set up training sessions to focus on specific areas that may be needed by practice employees. For example, you may want to train the phone center staff on messages and tasks but exclude other EMR features. Customized training sessions usually are the responsibility of the practice. *TIP:* Consider using a core team of clinical staff to develop the key training areas and train your staff on the specific items they need for their jobs.

Practice Procedures—EMR users should be trained on the EMR in light of the practice setups, templates and procedures. Practice procedures may include the various policies and workflows that have been designed by the practice to capitalize on the EMR. Practice procedure training may be built around practice-focused training on how to use the EMR. Indeed, practice procedures are the product of your workflow design and the various decisions that drive the EMR setup.

The actual training process may be staged to support the various stages of your EMR implementation. The following steps should be considered in developing your own training strategy:

Train super users—Super users training will be conducted by the vendor and cover all system features and capabilities. Super users are expected to serve the role of subject matter experts on the use and management of the EMR. Ideally, all users should have easy access to a super user. You may identify a super user for each location and/or department.

Develop practice training materials—Practice training materials allow you to focus on the specific strategies and setups of the EMR for your practice. This also allows you to integrate the training on the system with training staff on your own procedures, templates and setups. Training on practice procedures and practice training materials also support several HIPAA standards.

Train test and setup support staff—Additional staff can be used to support the system setup and testing process. For example, medical records staff can be used to test scanning options and clinical staff can be used to test templates and clinical documentation screens.

Identify training packages by role—Training all users on all aspects of the EMR will take a long time and provide many users with information that they will never use. Using the role definitions that drive the security setup, end users should be scheduled for training packages. The training packages should address the specific needs of each role.

Develop training plan—The end user training plan should train users for the work to be done in the current implementation step. The training should take place as close to the Go Live date for that particular function. For example, medical record training on scanning should be done immediately before scanning of medical records begins.

Train end users—End user training should take place as close to Go Live for the user as possible. For example, phone staff may train on messages immediately before they start using the EMR to log calls. End user training should include use of the workstation or tablet that will be used by the trainee. Note that end users may go through several training sequences as you expand the use of the system. For example, you may start off with imaging, move to workflow, proceed with charting and complete with order management. *TIP:* Remember that training classes should immediately precede actual use of the EMR. Otherwise the training effort will be a waste of time since most people will not remember how to use the system after a few weeks of inactivity.

Training practice staff on the EMR is an ongoing effort that will continue past EMR activation. Also, new employees will need to be fully trained on using the system. Current employees will need supplemental training on features that they have not used as well as changes to how the practice is making adjustments to EMR use. The EMR implementation effort allows the practice to set up the training materials and programs that will insure that the EMR usage is maintained according to the practice design as well as allow for evolving changes to meet practice needs and challenges (see Table 9.9).

TABLE 9.9

BASIC IMPLEMENTATION PLAN	STATUS	ASSIGNED TO	START	END	COMMENT
ADMINSTRATIVE					
1. Complete EMR implementation team.					
2. Kick-off meeting with vendor.					
POLICIES					
3. Establish a retention policy for scanned charts and originals that are scanned into the EMR.					
4. Establish policies and procedures for audit and quality assurance activities using the EMR.					
WORKFLOW AND PROCEDURE					
5. Develop EMR medical record workflow.					
6. Review EMR workflow flow charts with EMR project team.					
7. Develop detailed EMR procedures documents.					
TECHNOLOGY UPGRADES					
FACILITIES					
8. Upgrade the computer room for the EMR computer servers as well as existing equipment.					
9. Establish a training room with several workstations and wireless network access.					
COMMUNICATIONS					
10. Install wireless network equipment at practice sites.					
11. Test connectivity between tablets and wireless network at all appropriate areas.					
12. Evaluate intra-office and interoffice communications.					
SERVERS					
13. Install EMR servers.					
WORKSTATIONS/TABLETS					
14. Identify users needing tablets for wireless access.					

BASIC IMPLEMENTATION PLAN	STATUS	ASSIGNED TO	START	END	COMMENT
15. Identify current workstations that will need access to EMR.					
16. Identify, order and install new workstations that will be needed to support EMR.					
SCANNERS					
17. Complete inventory of all locations requiring small, medium and heavy-duty EMR scanner service.					
18. Install a testing scanner in medical records.					
19. Install all scanners and test with EMR.					
PRINTERS					
20. Complete inventory of new printers needed for EMR.					
21. Order printers.					
22. Install printers and test with EMR.					
CLINICAL CONTENT SETUP					
23. Compile samples of existing clinical forms, letters and reports.					
24. Map existing forms and reports to EMR clinical content and EMR setup.					
25 Arrange for training to support the EMR design.					
26. Analyze EMR setups, features and clinical content in light of practice forms and flow-sheets.					
27. Design and implement EMR setups.					
28. Test EMR setups.					
INTERFACES AND OTHER ISSUES					
29. Establish EMR report and production schedule.					
30. Implement interface between PMS and EMR.					

BASIC IMPLEMENTATION PLAN	STATUS	ASSIGNED TO	START	END	COMMENT
31. Test the interface between PMS and EMR.					
MASTER FILES					
32. Compile list of master file and information requirements For EMR.					
33. Analyze key master files issues and strategies for EMR.					
34. Collect EMR master file source information.					
35. Conduct training on EMR master file entry and setup.					
36. Enter EMR master file information into EMR.					
DATA CONVERSION					
37. Test scanning strategies and procedures with existing paper charts.					
38. Develop scanning procedures, triggers and strategies for the paper charts.					
39. Develop procedures for incoming faxes and mail that is loaded into the EMR.					
TRAINING					
40. Identify training team for EMR system administration, operations and production.					
41. Identify EMR training packages.					
42. Group staff into EMR roles for training staff.					
43. Train installation team on EMR.					
44. Develop practice-specific training materials for EMR and practice procedures.					
45. Train staff on master files.					
46. Train "train-the-trainer staff" for EMR workflow and charting.					
47. Train remaining staff on EMR in coordination with activation activities.					

BASIC IMPLEMENTATION PLAN	STATUS	ASSIGNED TO	START	END	COMMENT
48. Train medical record staff on the scanning of paper medical records.					
ACTIVATION					
49. Establish a chart disposition strategy for scanned charts.					
50. Set up production for chart scanning to work ahead of daily appointments.					
51. Initially load the PMS demographic information and scheduling information needed for Go Live.					
52. Establish computer operations, production scheduling and operational standards to support EMR.					
53. Initiate EMR audit support and tracking.					
54. Initiate use of the EMR.					

Activating an EMR

Once your practice starts moving to activate your EMR, expect some personnel and logistic issues. In some cases, staff and even doctors will leave a practice, protesting they "do not want to be computer operators." Some practices have experienced passive-aggressive behavior and sabotage. For example, doctors and employees may note that the EMR is slower that their paper-based process before they even fully use the system. You may even start questioning the value of the entire process.

The EMR will challenge employees who just do not like change. Some staff members will be afraid that they will lose their jobs or their influence. Other staff members may have years of time working with the paper record and be skeptical of the new EMR. Concern with job loss can be particularly acute in the most affected departments, such as medical records and transcription. Changes in staffing levels may be handled through normal attrition. In any case, don't expect to see job savings until several months after the EMR is activated. Indeed, most practices will experience greater expenses in the first transition year than the last non-EMR year. After the transition, you will be able to gauge the full effect and reap the benefits of the EMR.

EMR activation requires a massive change to every process and procedure. Know that the transfer of years of data and experience from the current records to an EMR is not accomplished in a day or two. The activation of the EMR requires a clear plan, commitment to the project and ability to address issues, because unexpected problems will arise in the middle of this massive change. For example, if patient flow depends on the EMR, then lapses in recording patient status or not checking the workflow screen on a constant basis will disrupt operations and frustrate everyone. EMR activation also requires patience and a focus on working out these problems.

Your activation strategy must consider the various factors and dynamics of the project as well as the need to complete the project. Activate the EMR only when your practice is ready. However, you need to move the project along at an even pace to complete activation in a manageable timeframe. The transition period accompanied by partial EMR use is complex and expensive to manage. For example, you have to pay for the management of paper records as well as the EMR during the transition period. As significant, maintaining a complete medical record may require addition efforts depending on your activation strategy.

In many cases, EMR activation is not so much an event, but a process. Depending on a wide array of issues, you may have various staff members using the EMR for work that is still paper based in other practice areas. For example, physician champions may be charting patient visits using the EMR, but medical records may still maintain the paper medical chart. Surviving and completing such transitions is the key to the activation process. Your practice, doctors, and staff will have to manage a number of transitions to complete the activation of the EMR. Some of these transitions will increase the workload of the practice, require additional resources, and frustrate everyone. However, coping with the changes during the transition is the only way to successfully activate and deploy the EMR. If you have a plan that the organization is behind, and you have the right product, then the process needed to implement the EMR should be allowed to proceed with the understanding that implementation is a complex and disruptive process. The successful completion of the activation process requires good management and commitment to the EMR strategy—throughout your organization.

ACTIVATION STRATEGIES

The activation of an EMR challenges the most capable staff and physicians. To succeed, you need to insure that all relevant doctors and staff understand their role and how you will activate the EMR. EMR activation can be based on any one of several strategies. Some vendors are very committed to one strategy, while others defer to the practice for the strategy and process. All EMR strategies consist of various groupings and orders of the following EMR capabilities:

Paperless chart stage—Some practices go through a paperless chart phase before they commence charting patient visits into the EMR. The paperless chart phase involves scanning the paper chart and providing access to the patient chart through the scanned EMR images. New information is entered on a paper form and the paper form is scanned into the EMR. The practice must deal with the EMR to access information but use paper to record information. In some cases, the paperless chart is the final end point of the EMR effort. The physicians will nonetheless benefit from immediate access to the patient chart instead of waiting for the paper record.

Charge and limited clinical information entry—The physicians and staff will use the EMR workstations and/or personal digital assistants to enter charge and limited EMR information, such as prescriptions, allergies and other basic patient data. Charges are passed to the PMS for billing. In some cases, you can also dictate directly into a transcription tool that is part of the EMR. For some practices, these functions are the end of their EMR effort. Some EMR vendors sell this limited set of capabilities as a "starting point" to move to the full EMR at a later date.

Doctor charting—Practices may start use of the EMR with selected patients and doctors to chart patient visits at time of service. Selected doctors will use the EMR to collect discrete information to document a patient visit while the patient is being served. For example, the nurse may enter vitals into the EMR record, but the doctor may dictate the assessment and plan. Using charting at time of service, the doctor enters information into the EMR and uses the EMR to calculate the E&M code for the visit. If the practice is not paperless, the chart record is printed from the EMR and filed in the patient's paper chart. *Note* that all doctors will not start charting at the same time, and will not start charting for all patients at once. Typically, the doctor will start charting for patient visits that they feel comfortable with. For example, a doctor may start with a single patient each day for a specific type of visit (for instance, flu, simple problem) and proceed to increase their EMR charting for all patients with the selected problem and then adding additional problems and conditions. The physician should practice with a previous visit, role play with staff, and/or shadow a patient visit to insure that he is ready to chart at time of service. The early-adopter physicians may mentor other doctors and users as they start using the EMR to chart patient visits. ***CAUTION:*** Doctors should cautiously move into charting with the EMR. Otherwise, they are putting too much pressure on themselves and the practice which could increase the chance of failure.

Transcription into the EMR—Dictated notes are entered into the EMR by a transcriptionist. The notes are saved in the EMR and the EMR may be used to coordinate review and distribution. If the practice is not paperless, the transcription may be printed and filed in the patient chart. For many practices, using the EMR to manage transcription offers an easy way to build up patient information in anticipation of implementing the EMR. Indeed, you may start using the transcription module to build up patient clinical content long before you are charting patient visits in the EMR. Immediate access to patient dictation is a significant benefit for practices that use dictation. ***TIP:*** EMR based access to transcription files is more effective and secure than transcription files that are generally available on a network server or stored on the transcriptionist's workstation.

Order entry and management—Doctors and clinical staff record and manage testing and treatment orders through the EMR. Orders are entered and assigned to the appropriate department. The order is managed by the department and the status of the order may be entered into the EMR. Note that the actual results may be managed through the paper record or through the EMR. The EMR offers the added benefit of being able to identify incomplete or pending services or treatments.

EMR Order tracking is far superior to having outstanding items buried in a paper record or on a supplemental log. This capability can help the practice serve patients and follow-up on the doctor's advice. For example, the appointment clerk could check for outstanding tests or services when scheduling a patient.

Prescription entry—Prescriptions are entered into the EMR and produced for the patient. Prescriptions may be printed, faxed and/or electronically submitted to a designated pharmacy. In some cases, prescription writing is a separate module that may be used outside of implementing a complete EMR. Note that many practices have been disappointed with the final results of only entering prescriptions and not implementing an EMR. Some practices believe that they are only doing the pharmacy's data entry and seeing few benefits for the practice. Indeed, stand alone prescription systems do not necessarily save any work or time, since the prescription is still recorded in the patient note, prescription log and other documents.

Workflow—Practice staff and doctors use the EMR to manage patient workflow and issues. Patient messages, office issues, prescription refills and other items are entered and tracked in the EMR. The doctors and clinical staff access their assigned items, but need access to the paper chart to address the issue or answer the question. The resolution of the item is noted in the EMR. If the paper chart is still in use, the workflow items may be printed out and filed in the paper chart. EMR-based workflow tools will help management track items and insure that patient issues are addressed in a timely basis.

In some cases, vendors will group various capabilities together based on the structure of their system, your practice situation or any number of factors. For example, some vendors insist on charge entry and prescription writing for their initial EMR functions.

The activation sequence and what is included in each activation group should be seriously reviewed and considered before you move forward. **TIP**: Be especially careful to manage the implementation process on your schedule and not necessarily the "sunny day" schedule proposed by other parties. You need to be realistic about the practical effect of your activation strategy and steps. The various transition phases that are determined by your strategy will not necessarily save you time or money from the first step of your transition process. Converting to an EMR requires a lot of flexibility, enthusiasm, and commitment. You also need to be patient through the transition steps to complete the implementation process and take advantage of your investment.

For example, you need to let your key users digest the training on the EMR before you commence end-user training. Some vendors propose schedules that assume your newly trained key users return from training as experts. They rarely are that quickly. Additionally, you must be certain that a reliable patient medical record is available throughout the process. Split medical records with some information in the paper record and other information in the EMR can expose the practice to HIPAA compliant issues as well as inhibit patient care.

Using some features and adding additional capabilities over time is an excellent way to transition to the EMR. However, the transition period should be as short as possible due to the complexity of managing both the paper and computerized patient records. For example, charting patient visits on the EMR and printing for a paper record could create medical record continuity problems. Too many practices fall into the trap of implementing a few capabilities and stopping. A partially implemented EMR could be very dangerous and expensive. Your staff and doctors can only go so long with having to deal with patient information split between the EMR and your paper records. Indeed, some practices get to a point where they give up and go back to their paper records. The key to success is moving quickly through the implementation process and avoid sitting in transition for too long. For example, a scanned medical record may be more difficult for many doctors than the original paper record. However, order entry, charting and prescriptions will ultimately make things easier. If the practice is stuck in the scanned record mode for too long, the physicians and staff may get frustrated.

ACTIVATION READINESS

Now you're just about ready use the EMR in your practice. To manage and control the process, you need to insure that you have the resources and support structure in place to deal with this dramatic and challenging step. This includes:

Physician champions—The biggest barrier to charting at time of service is clinical content. The verification and testing of clinical content is one challenge, but reaching a comfort level with the clinical content will make the difference for physicians. Your practice needs at least one physician champion to start EMR use. Some practices have several physician champions to cover various practice areas. The physician(s) must be willing to put up with the inevitable start up issues and adjustments. Of course, the more testing and training, the fewer problems. Physicians involved in the testing process should continue to use the charting tool to maintain training continuity and build experience. Physicians and staff need to practice documenting patient visits and using the EMR a number of times before they are ready to use the EMR for patient service. You may even consider generating the clinical record to be filed in your paper chart (to adequately control and maintain the designated record set). Physicians should be encouraged to use the charting tool to gain confidence and experience. These same physicians will become the mentors to the other doctors.

Employee readiness—The entire practice staff must be fully trained. Staff should be told to support new users of the EMR. Training materials, guides and workflow issues should be tested and ready for activation. A sufficient number of employees should have been involved in system setup and testing to provide a good base for activation. Immediately before activation, all of the remaining users will be trained on the EMR. As previously noted, such training should occur immediately before the user starts using the EMR—so the training is fresh in their minds. ***TIP:*** Make sure you take advantage of operational offices and doctors as part of your training process. For example, doctors who are using the EMR already could be mentors for doctors who are still training on EMR use. Clinical staff could be rotated into the locations that are already using the EMR prior to their EMR Go Live.

Activation meetings—As the activation date approaches, you need to monitor progress across a wide range of activities. Hold meetings with key staff across these activities. These allow you to allocate resources and make decisions to address issues as well as monitor their activities in preparing for EMR activation. These meetings should focus on practice readiness and critical path items to support the activation process. For example, the activation process may require the contemporaneous completion of user training and patient demographic loading from the PMS. Note that delays in the activation process will become more costly and disruptive as the project proceeds. For example, delay of the entire project is less disruptive than a delay between the start of scanning of medical records and the charting of patient visits.

Onsite support—Dedicated support staff should be positioned at each site in your practice as the EMR is activated. Support resources include vendor trainers, super users, managers and supervisors. Respond to user needs and issues quickly to get users over the initial startup challenges. For example, users may not be familiar with how to document a side issue that is outside the standard clinical data supported by the EMR. Make sure that each user has immediate access to a support person to help him through problems or issues. Additional support may be available by having software and hardware vendor staff onsite, as well as pulling other resources from various practice units. For example, you may place your computer support and billing office staff to provide additional support during the initial startup phase.

Key contacts—Keep a list of key contacts for hardware, software and support on call to immediately address any last minute challenges and items. You also need management ready to address procedural issues that may crop up during the initial system startup. For example, you may fall behind in scanning patient records for appointments.

Mentoring—In addition to training staff, the doctors and clinicians should be supported by mentors. The mentoring program should pair key users and computer savvy staff with less confident users. The mentoring process is critical to allow users to be served and not overwhelm the practice support staff during the activation and first few weeks of EMR use.

Your activation steps may follow several strategies. Some practices gradually adopt various EMR components on the way to full EMR use. Other practices implement several pieces at a time leading up to full EMR activation. After you have chosen your activation sequence, your activation plan should generally include the following tasks:

Verify policies and procedures—This insures that written training materials and procedures are properly documented. Be sure to check that users have current versions of your documents and *not* draft copies used during testing and setup.

Complete staff training—By the time you are ready to activate the EMR, a number of staff members should be fairly comfortable with the EMR. However, you may want to do some focused training on the use of the EMR in production mode that may differ from the training and testing to date. New user training should occur as close as possible to the date the user starts EMR use. Delays could result in lost knowledge and continuity problems.

Verify hardware operations—All hardware devices should be verified and staged for use by employees and doctors. Before activation, the various devices should be checked for access to the EMR and system facilities. For example, you need to verify that each tablet can correctly communicate with the wireless network. In some cases, hardware and software setups to back up training will not support the active system. For example, some EMRs have a test database that is actually maintained through a system initialization file. You should also verify that you can quickly and effectively respond to specific hardware problems and even failures. For example, you should have a person at each location that can swap out a problem piece of equipment and/or resolve a problem connecting to the EMR.

Complete EMR setup—The EMR setup should be completed. The physician super-users should verify that they have completed the setup of the clinical content. For example, some EMR setups that were staged in the test database must be transferred or entered in the production database. Note that the transferred clinical setups should be checked and verified to insure that the production database works. *CAUTION:* Some EMR products do not allow you to copy setup information from the test system to the production system: you have to reenter the setup information in the production system. Other EMR products do not even have test systems.

Initial load of demographic data—Prior to using the EMR, you need to load the demographic information that will be associated with the clinical data. Ideally, you should load these data electronically from your PMS. You need to activate the interface between the PMS and EMR systems and verify that the entire demographic database is available through the EMR. *TIP*: Verify the total number of demographic records and test search patient appointments for the first day. Do a test to verify that demographic changes are being passed from the PMS to the EMR. The verification process is needed to check that the production database (and not the test system) contains the appropriate information.

Initial load of appointment information—As noted with the demographic information, the appointment information must be initially loaded into the production database. You should also verify that the PMS is sending appointment updates to the production database and not the test database. *CAUTION:* Make sure to check the interface for patient checkin in the PMS (where applicable) to make sure the EMR workflow indicates the patients are available to be seen on a real time basis.

Initial load of electronic clinical data—A variety of clinical data may be loaded into the EMR before activation. Electronic clinical date may be available from diagnostic equipment and lab information systems that are interfaced with the EMR. Additional information sources include transcription files and information from the PMS. The electronic information should be loaded into the EMR according to the interface plan. Note that you may only download data based on a trigger (e.g., patient appointment) or all data from a selected period. **CAUTION:** Be sure to check the implications of information that is electronically loaded into the EMR with the same information that may be scanned from the patient's paper record into the EMR.

Initial load of paper clinical data—To activate the EMR, you need to provide the information needed from the paper medical record. Some practices continue use of the paper record during the transition period. Others practices scan the paper record into the EMR and use the EMR as the sole access point and repository of clinical information. The scanning process should be structured to work ahead of the appointment schedule in much the same way that you may pull charts three days before the appointment. Additional charts will be processed to support phone calls, hospital procedures and other clinical services. Depending on your activation strategy (see Chapter 9—Implementing an EMR), the initial load of paper clinical data may include a summarization of the paper record into the EMR.

A timeline for two stage EMR activation is presented at the end of this chapter (see Figure 10.1). The timeline initially implements a paperless chart and workflow features. During the initial stage, physicians would document patient visits on paper or use dictation that would be saved in the EMR. A few weeks are allowed for adjusting to the scanning and workflow use as well as allowing for final testing of the clinical charting capability. The second phase activates clinical charting by physicians in two groups. Note that in both cases, the practice is counting on staff involved in setup and testing to provide a basic level of experience and support for new users. The other benefit of this strategy is that the setup and testing team understands the strategy and rational for the EMR setups used.

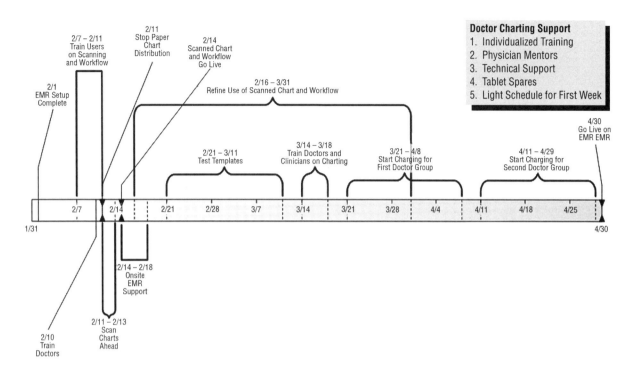

FIGURE 10.1—*Sample Activation Timeline*

)

Supporting an EMR

Your practice has gone through a process that included reworking your operations, making policies and staging the EMR. The EMR implementation effort involved everyone in your practice and affected every patient. To preserve the value of your EMR investment, you need a multifaceted approach to control and monitor use. Protecting the EMR requires technical, organizational and management strategies. As an added bonus, some of these strategies will help you comply with various HIPAA security and privacy standards.

SUPPORT POLICIES

Your support program should be guided and empowered by practice policies designed to enforce procedures and training standards as well as structure changes. Unilateral decisions to change processes, use or system setups undermine your clinical documentation and management of the practice. For example, failure to follow initial intake information templates could lead to additional work for the doctor and a lower E&M code, costing you entitled reimbursement. The support policies should guide doctors as well as staff. Basic policies include:

> **Employee standards**—The practice may choose to develop a general guideline for new employees. The guideline may include the level of computer competency as well as a pre-employment test on basic computer skills. Current employees should meet an escalating level of knowledge based on the needs of the practice and their position. For example, a phone operator will need additional training on demographics to staff the check-in desk. Employee standards should reflect these new needs. For example, suspended employees should not have access to the EMR.

Clinical charting standards—To support the clinical standards developed in the EMR implementation process, your chief medical officer should establish a clinical practices committee. The clinical practices committee will monitor use of charting standards as well as guide enhancements to the documentation standards. The committee will review, approve, design and test changes to templates and EMR setups. The clinical charting standards committee may also review compliance with the clinical standards by doctors and clinical staff. Some practices establish documentation standards that doctors must use to insure consistency and mitigate clinical and treatment risks. For example, a clinical treatment standard that included a certain test on a periodic basis would be used by all doctors.

Training standards—Establish training standards for doctors and staff. The training standards will specify the functional requirements for each role in the practice. For example, billing staff may be trained on accessing and printing medical record portions. You should also consider incentives to encourage employees to raise their knowledge and skills. ***TIP***: Establish a bonus plan for employees who reach a certain level of EMR proficiency.

EMR access and use—Practice management should establish the access and use standards for the practice. These standards should meet the HIPAA privacy and security guidelines. EMR access should be clearly defined for each employee role. The policy should specify the penalties for violations. The EMR access and use policies may include audit requirements and rules for reporting compliance issues to management. For example, an audit procedure may verify the "need-to-know" standard for selected patients and employees on a periodic basis. Violations may be reported to management, perhaps, on a monthly basis.

Performance monitoring and problem resolution—The practice should establish a mechanism to monitor EMR performance and problems. The policy may require reporting on interruptions, problems and issues on a monthly basis. The management oversight will insure that key issues are addressed at the executive level and appropriate communications are maintained with vendors and staff on use issues. This mechanism will assure management oversight of this increasingly important function.

TRAINING PROGRAM

Training and retraining users insures they are fully informed and adequately knowledgeable on how to use the EMR. The practice should schedule training programs to introduce new users and update current users on EMR use. You training program is part of your HIPAA privacy and security compliance efforts. The training program will insure that the system is used consistently throughout the practice according to the established policies and procedures.

Be sure the training program has written documentation and/or manuals. The written materials can include screen shots and instructions to guide use of the system. The documentation should reflect your specific procedures as well as how you set up the EMR. For example, you may establish new department breakdowns and roles to capitalize on instantaneous access to the patient chart. The training materials should focus on your practice. Don't delve into non-relevant topics. For example, a urology practice may exclude training on the use of the EMR growth charts.

You can undertake an elaborate document or piece together information from copies of manual pages. In any case, the training manual should focus on how the system is used in the practice and your expectations. For example, you may include lists of your document types and what documents are classified for each of your document types. The document could include routing and priority standards for each document type. Such priority standards could be used by practice managers to focus resources on an operational basis as well as monitor average response times for management tracking.

New employees should be trained on the features that are relevant to their job according to user roles. Train new employees as soon as they come on board. Ideally, each new employee should be assigned a mentor to insure that the new employee adapts to the practice's EMR methods using your own procedures. *TIP*: Use the audit records to monitor new employee performance and double-check their work. Note that new employees can be an excellent source of ideas and suggestions.

Retrain current employees on a periodic basis. The retraining effort should include a review of the EMR features and procedures used in their areas. Such training could be conducted by employees who have demonstrated a superior command of the product. Retraining insures that all employees are using the same processes on a consistent basis. Employees who have difficulty using the EMR within the established procedure framework should receive supplemental training. For example, a user who documents phone messages in a patient note instead of a patient task would receive supplemental training in both areas.

On occasion, you will need to train all current users on a change to the system or a new software release. The training program should be designed to cover all employees in a compressed timeframe. The updated process should be supported by appropriate training materials and procedure documentation. *TIP*: Conduct the training in a room that includes the equipment used in the practice.

HARDWARE AND SOFTWARE SUPPORT

Supporting an EMR requires an ongoing hardware and software maintenance effort. The entire technology base should be continually reviewed to insure it meets your needs, and that your system evolves to meet the changes to your practice. In too many cases, the completion of EMR implementation leads to complacency. Lack of attention to your system can cause troubles.

Your system is subject to changes due to business, industry, management and clinical issues. For example, new diagnostic equipment may speed the intake of patients requiring a frequently administered test. A new office, new service offering, changes in your patient base, and/or additional doctors could affect your technology needs. Additional clinical services may require more clinical content that the EMR doesn't have.

Even if the EMR contains appropriate clinical content, the clinical content has to be tested by the practice. Additional offices and users could exceed the communication capacity that was designed for the system. Additional users and increased volume could exceed the designed capacity of the system or consume disk space at a more rapid rate. Although growth and changes are not a problem, the EMR must be enhanced and expanded to meet the changes in your practice. Otherwise, the EMR could fall into disuse and risk failure. For example, the new doctors may use another system because the practice's EMR lacks support for their subspecialty. Multiple EMRs in a single practice is costly and harms coordination.

Any strategic decision should include an analysis of the technology impact. The existing technology should be reviewed in light of the projected change. For example, new diagnostic equipment may be able to directly interface with the EMR to speed patient services. Yet, introduction of mid-level providers enabled by the EMR may increase the user count and the load on the system.

The projected changes should be analyzed to insure that the servers, communications and software setups will be able to support the changes. For example, new services may require a new department setup instead of crowding patient flow and messages into an existing department. Additional services may necessitate the review of classifications and management structures to avoid the growth of "miscellaneous" classifications throughout the system. Note that system enhancements should be completed before you need them and *not* in the middle of a performance crisis.

Regardless of the expense and effort, you cannot cost effectively eliminate the possibility that the EMR may fail. You can invest in redundant hardware, uninterruptible power supplies and a host of options and still experience a failure. On the other hand, some practices go for years without a disruption. As a matter of prudence, assume that you will lose access to the EMR for 1–2 days/year. The loss may be due to a communication problem, power failure, hardware failure and/or a software issue, but you should be prepared to get by for a day or two without the EMR. *TIP*: Design your system to tolerate problems, monitor your system to catch issues before you experience a system failure, have a plan for operating in the event of a failure and be prepared to quickly address failures.

Effective hardware support begins with good system design. We have previously discussed a number of strategies and options to consider in your initial purchase. However, your hardware base will change over time due to expansion of the practice, new offices and services, device replacements and hardware capacity. Manage your hardware situation by reviewing each change for:

> **Strategic hardware and software support**—Changes to the hardware and software should be completed within the structure of a strategic plan. For example,

piecemeal workstation upgrades could lead to continuing disruptions to the entire system. If you need more powerful workstations, you should plan ahead to insure new workstations are based on the evolving requirements and not the baseline needs of the current software. And you can avoid separate virus protection purchases for each workstation by employing a virus-detection system on a server. Backup device planning should be based on strategic needs and not the minimum requirements. A number of practices have had to suddenly contend with the inability to back up their systems overnight. Switching to a weekly backup leaves the practice seriously exposed to a tragic loss of information.

EMRs will consume substantially more space in a much shorter time than anything the practice has previously encountered. Diagnostic images and scanned medical charts can consume more space in a day than your may need for a year of financial transactions. A number of practices have had to suddenly contend with the inability to back up their system overnight. The backup equipment and strategy should accommodate complete backups of the entire database on a periodic basis as well as interim partial backups. For example, some EMRs ask you to backup every 30–60 minutes.

Security Issues and Enhancements—Monitoring security issues and challenges is a continuing process. Any new hardware and software should be reviewed in light of your security and privacy standards. New hardware should be set up to support the existing security standards including communications, virus protection, access codes and automatic logging off. New software should be reviewed to insure that the appropriate security features and options are used. For example, you may need to review your security access strategy by user role. Be especially careful to check that intermediate files containing patient information are kept on unsecured devices. For example, print images, intermediate image files from diagnostic devices and workstation-based documents require cleanup and maintenance to assure confidentiality. On a periodic basis, you should review compliance with your security standards as well as any security problems. For example, firewall logs and software audit records should be reviewed on a periodic basis for security violations and intrusion attempts. In some cases, practices use a third-party systems' integrator to review the system logs and stability of the database on a periodic basis.

System access—An increasing number of healthcare organizations and vendors will seek to exchange data with your systems. You need to be extremely vigilant and skeptical to insure that you maintain the security of your systems. For example, a software vendor requested opening the firewall for easier access. The easier access for the vendor would have exposed the practice to computer attacks from other parties. In some cases, practices are giving access to EMR data for related providers and physicians. Note that such access may not be supported by your EMR product and could open your practice to security and privacy problems.

In some cases, you may get early warning of impending system problems. Intermittent interruptions, slow performance and other problems may be early signs of a larger system problem. To avoid these issues, the practice should monitor performance and check hardware components on a periodic basis. For example, some systems require maintenance tasks to recapture disk space. You should also monitor hardware for problems that may indicate the end of the useful life of system components. System components should be replaced before and not because of catastrophic failures.

If your EMR is at a secured hosting site or you use an Application Service Provider (ASP), you should conduct periodic reviews of any changes at the site as well as examine any interruptions that required the use of backup systems and communication links. A periodic meeting with the ASP representative and appropriate reports will allow you to make sure you are protected.

On a periodic basis, you will need to upgrade your software. For example, your EMR vendor may release a new upgrade to support additional features and address problems. In many cases, vendors will only support a previous version or two of the product. Ideally, you should wait to install the upgrade until you have verified that other practices are successfully using the new version. You should insure that the system includes all of the functionality and modules that you are currently using. For example, you may have to wait until the vendor includes a module you use in the next product upgrade.

You should also verify that your hardware and system software will support the new version of your EMR. For example, a new version may require additional disk space for a new access and audit log. In other cases, the vendor may have changed the minimum hardware requirements. If you are sure that the update is stable, then you should perform a test conversion or installation and verify the update works. Having completed testing, you need to coordinate training on the new update with its planned installation of live data. Note that some system upgrades are easily installed with your current data, while others may require conversion of your current data. In any event, make sure you always maintain a backup of the pre-update system to allow you to fall back to the working system in the event of a problem.

You should also be careful to validate the amount of time needed for the conversion to the upgrade. In some cases, upgrades require a weekend conversion. The actual conversion time will depend on the complexity of the upgrade, the speed of your hardware and the size of your database.

Disaster Recovery

In the unlikely event of a failure, you should have a remediation and recovery plan for various potential problems. The plan should have specific instructions to address various system failures, including the full or partial loss of the EMR and localized loss of system access. For example, you may lose the ability to print anything from the EMR. The plan documentation should include a detailed explanation of the current system components and software. The plan should allow for continuing operations while you work on the problem.

In many cases, you may encounter a problem that increases the risk of a serious problem, but does not noticeably affect operations. For example, the failure of a communication line to an office that is closed for the day may go immediately unnoticed but is a sign of a serious problem. Address such issues with urgency. Practices often fail to fix the little problems until a big failure occurs. By proactively going after problems and monitoring system issues and performance, you may be able to resolve them before they cause disruptions.

Your remediation plan should include:

Notification protocols—Depending on the type of loss, your plan should indicate the various parties that should be notified. Practice management, key vendors and supervisors should be informed of the problem and status. Note the vendor response and monitor it. Throughout the crisis, practice staff and management should be updated on status and expected recovery.

Operational protocols—The operational strategy during the system loss should be documented and available to all employees. Employees should be periodically trained on the fall-back procedures. For example, paper flowsheets may be used during the loss to continue patient services. In cases where the hardware features fall-back options, you may need to scale back EMR use. For example, you may need to stop scanning from remote locations when you use a slower backup communications link to a remote office. Similarly, you may need to limit the number of users if a key server fails.

EMR recovery—Once the EMR is operational, the plan should specify how the information accumulated during the outage will be added to the EMR system. Verify that full operations are restored. Some outages may require staged activation of EMR components. For example, it may take longer to reestablish interfaces with diagnostic equipment than to restart the EMR.

Post-recovery review—After the problem has been resolved and the system has been restored, the problem and recovery activities should be reviewed to determine potential improvements to the plan and changes to avoid future problems. Such a review should be undertaken for unexpected situations and failures. For example, frequent disk failures could target what needs to be corrected to avoid future problems.

USER SUPPORT

To protect your EMR investment, you need to set up a structure that avoids "creeping disability." Creeping disability results from changes to meet evolving issues without fully evaluating the effects on the practice. Creeping disability also is caused by users abandoning the EMR for other solutions. For example, a doctor may start documenting patient visits using typed notes instead of templates and clinical content. Quality assurance reports and patient selection reports based on template information may not include patient notes. Employees who use their own task classification codes and priority flags will not be included in management reports and performance tracking.

In reality, your practice staff will know more about the EMR in your practice than your vendor after 3–6 months. Vendor support staff may not be familiar with the various setups and templates you use. You need to establish a process that insures that you control user support and maintain the value of your EMR investment. The support mechanism insures that you keep using the system as you designed and that the EMR evolves in a way that better serves your practice.

User support addresses user issues on a day-to-day basis. The best support structures provide immediate feedback to users who have a question or issue. Informal support structures may not produce resolutions. Indeed, the support structure helps the user but also enforces the practice's standards. User support requires a hierarchical approach that provides front-line support on a continuing basis that is backed by management strategies:

Front-line support—Each department and working area should have a "go to" person for daily support issues. The front-line support person should be knowledgeable in the EMR functions and practice procedures that are relevant to the department. The front-line support person should be able to perform basic troubleshooting on local hardware issues and to answer software questions. User issues and needs should get to super users or computer support through the front-line support person. The front-line support person insures that you make the best use of each level of staff to identify, address and resolve computer issues.

Super-user support—If a problem requires a change to the way you use the EMR or one of your procedures, the problem must be passed on to a super user. The practice managers or super users will be able to make decision on changes to the EMR use or practice procedures that can be applied to the entire practice. The super users should be able to look at the issue from a practice level. This helps to make sure changes that are helpful to one department will not create problems in another area. For example, scanning incoming clinical documents may complicate operations at the front desk but significantly eases clinical workflow.

Computer support—If the front-line support staff is unable to resolve a technical computer hardware or software issue, get the designated computer support person/staff involved. The computer support person/staff serves as the resident technical expert on the computer system as well as the point of contact with vendors on technical issues. In some cases, the practice staff includes a basic technical support person that is supplemented with an outside consultant or network support group. In other cases, practices employ a complete technical support team to administer the computer network and address technical issues. The practice computer support staff coordinates EMR server or application issues with the EMR vendor. Frequently, the application and procedure issues are managed by super users.

Regardless of how well you implemented the EMR, new issues and situations will evolve that will require adjustments and changes. The practice needs a mechanism to identify, analyze and resolve these issues. Your solution to evolving issues rests in the same structure you used to implement the system: your implementation team and super users.

Key EMR users should meet on a monthly basis to review EMR use and evolving issues. The purpose of the monthly EMR review meetings is to maintain the momentum of adaptation, and identify problems to fix. The meeting should identify the go-forward strategy for each problem. Issues may be solved through changes to procedures, adjustments to the system setups and/or changes to templates. In some cases, changes will require vendor enhancements. The monthly review meetings should consider a list of all outstanding issues. Report these issues to the practice management team.

Due to the number of users and the critical nature of the EMR, the practice should consider the use of automated support tools to log problems and provide assistance. The computer support software should allow designated users to log problems, as well as facilitate management and tracking of support issues by managers and designated IT staff. For example, you may want to know EMR problems by type and resolution. A number of products can support your practice computer support needs. DataTrack (www.magnosoft.biz) and Track-It (www.itsolutions.intuit.com) are examples of products that manage computer user support issues.

SYSTEM AUDIT PROCEDURES

In many systems, a variety of information is maintained behind the scenes to track user activities and system performance. Based on the information maintained by the EMR, you should conduct periodic audits of various system activities. System audit procedures will help you maintain practice performance and support users. System audit areas can include user activities, unauthorized activities by users and attempts to access the system by unauthorized users. Other audit procedures may track open clinical notes, incomplete tasks and overdue patient procedures. Hardware and network audits may analyze attacks on the firewall, virus attacks and events, quarantine files and failed exchanges among practice systems.

The system audit should include tracking of monthly activities and trend analysis. The system audit results should be reported to management.

APPENDIX

CCHIT (www.cchit.org) provides certification based on an analysis of electronic medical records. CCHIT measures products under a defined and published standard. The CCHIT status has been added to our vendor chart to identify those products that have met the CCHIT certification standard.

EMR Product	Contact Information (Company, Address, Phone, Website)	Number of Installations/ Company Founded	CCHIT Status	PMS Options	Key Clinical Areas
HEALTHMAT-ICS EMR (See Allscripts)	A⁴ HEALTH SYSTEMS - See Allscripts				
ABELMed PM - EMR Version 7.0	ABELSoft Corporation 3310 South Service Road Burlington, Ontario CANADA L7N 3M6 800-263-5104 www.ABELSoft.com	1977	Certified 10/23/06	ABELMed is a complete PMS and EMR product.	
AcerMed EMR 1.0	AcerMed, Inc. 135 Technology Dr., Suite #200 Irvine, CA 92618 800-841-0008/949-250-4410 www.acermed.com	56 Practices (New Product) 1987	Certified 10/23/06	AcerMed PM and Centricity PMS.	Pediatrics Orthopaedics
Accumedic's Electronic Medical Record Software	Accumedic Computer Sys., Inc. 11 Grace Ave. Suite 401 Great Neck, NY 11021 516-466-6800/800-765-9300 www.accumedic.com	1977	In Process	Accumed, EMDEON, Quic-DOC, Praxis EMR, ReDOC, HBOC STAR and any HL7 enabled EMR system.	
MedicsDoc-Assistant 3.0	AdvancedMD Software, Inc 11781 South Lone Peak Pkwy, Suite 110 Draper, UT 84020 801-984-9500 www.advancedmd.com	1,000 + Users 1999	Certified 1/29/07	AdvancedEMR in-cludes AdvancedMD.	
AllMeds EMR Version 7	AllMeds, Inc. 151 Lafayette Dr, Suite 401 Oak Ridge, TN 37830 888-343-MEDS www.allmeds.com	100+ Practices 1999	Certified 4/30/07	Interfaced with several PMS prod-ucts including Centricity PMS, and MISYS	Supports sev-eral specialties including ENT and Cardiology.
TouchWorks HER 11.0	Allscripts 222 Merchandise Mart Plaza Suite 2024 Chicago, IL 60654 800-654-0889 www.allscripts.com	150+ Practices	Certified 7/18/06	Partners with IDX	Supports a wide range of special-ties with the Medcin data-base.
HealthMatics HER 2006	Allscripts 5501 Dillard Drive Cary, NC 27518 888-672-3282 www.allscripts.com	1,300	Certified 7/18/06	Companion PMS with HealthMatics NtierPrise. Estab-lished interfaces with many PMS products.	Primary Care and Selected Specialties

Continued

EMR Product	Contact Information (Company, Address, Phone, Website)	Number of Installations/ Company Founded	CCHIT Status	PMS Options	Key Clinical Areas
Alteer Office™ Alteer Corporation	4 Venture, Suite 100 Irvine, CA 92618 949-789-0500 www.alteer.com	400+ Practices 1996		Integrated EMR/PMS	
Clarus® - Clinical Documentation	American HealthNet 2110 S. 169th Plaza Omaha, NE 68130 402-733-2700/800-745-4712 www.americanhealthnet.com	6 Hospitals 1980		EMPI – (Enterprise Master Patient Index) HL7 Compliant	Hospitals, Clinics, Orthopaedics.
Electronic Patient Chart	American Medical Software 1180 S. State Hwy. 157 PO Box 236 Edwardsville, IL 62025 800.423.8836 www.americanmedical.com	2,500 Practices 1984		Companion PMS with PMP Practice Management PLUS	Primary, Internal, Surgical practices.
Intuition EMR	AMICAS, Inc. 20 Guest Street Boston, MA 02135-2040 800-490-8465 www.amicas.com/home.asp				
Amicore Clinical Management	Amicore 200 Minuteman Rd. Andover, MA 01810 978-691-3400 www.amicore.com	2001 – Acquired by Misys in 2006		Companion PMS with Amicore Practice Management	
AmkaiCharts	Amkai, Inc. 255 Bank Street FL 2B Waterbury, CT 06702 203-755-5151/866-265-2434 www.amkai.net	26 Centers 3000 users 1984		AmkaiOffice AdvantX, SIS, Vision via XML and HL7	Ambulatory Surgery Centers
Electronic Clinical Record	Anasazi Software 9831 S. 51st Street Suite C117 Phoenix, AZ 85044 800-651-4411 www.anasazisoftware.com	1993		Integrated with other Anasazi Systems.	Behavioral Healthcare
athenaClinicals ™ 0.15	athenahealth, Inc. 311 Arsenal Street Watertown, MA 02472 888-652-8200 www.athenahealth.com	20 Practices 1997	Certified 4/30/07	AthenaHealth	Anesthesia, Occupational Health

Continued

EMR Product	Contact Information (Company, Address, Phone, Website)	Number of Installations/ Company Founded	CCHIT Status	PMS Options	Key Clinical Areas
Elysium EMR	Axolotl Corp. 800 El Camino Real W., Ste. 150 Mountain View, CA 94040 650-964-1100/888-296-5685 www.axolotl.com	12,500 Practices 1995		Many PMS connections through HL7 Compliant Repository	Primary Care
PrognoCIS 1.81	BizMatics, Inc. 20863 Stevens Creek Blvd. Suite 540 Cupertino, CA 95014 866-873-3030 www.bizmaticsinc.com	2002	Certified 4/30/07	Easy integration with many clinical systems through HL7.	
E-Paperless EMR V2.01	BMD Services 5201 Hwy 6, Suite 500 Missouri City, TX 77459 281-208-5403 www.bmdservices.net		Certified 4/30/07	E-Paperless Practice V2.01	
Physician's Solution 3.0	BLM MedRecords Alert LLC		Certified 4/30/2007		
Bond Clinician EHR 2006	Bond Technologies 3903 Northdale Boulevard Suite 115 West Tampa, FL 33624 866.792.6900 www.bondclinician.com	25+ Practices 2004	Certified 10/23/06	Integrated with Bond PMS.	Ambulatory Surgery Centers, Anesthesiology, Cardiology, Dermatology, Endocrinology, Gastroenterology, Nephrology, Neurology and Neurosurgery, Obstetrics and Gynecology, Oncology, Ophthalmology, Orthopedic, Otolaryngology, Pediatrics, Plastic Surgery, Primary Care, Pulmonary, Sleep Medicine, Urology

Continued

EMR Product	Contact Information (Company, Address, Phone, Website)	Number of Installations/ Company Founded	CCHIT Status	PMS Options	Key Clinical Areas
PEARL EMR 6.0	Business Computer Applications, Inc. 2002 Perimeter Summit Blvd Suite 880 Atlanta, GA 30319 800-648-1555 www.bca.us	1997	Certified 4/30/07	HL7 compliant	Federally Qualified Health Centers, Correctional Health.
Cabinet NG SAFE	Cabinet NG, Inc. 9668 Madison, Suite 100 Madison, AL 35758 256-256-0460/800-621-6501 www.cabinetng.com	100+ Practices		Supports PMS interfaces through HL7, ODBC, and SQL.	Document Management Product
Accelerator Graphical Health Record 4.111	Catalis, Inc. 916 S. Capital of Texas Hwy. Austin, TX 78746 888-241-1325 www.theCatalis.com	2005	Certified 1/29/07		
PowerChart 2005.02	Cerner Corporation 2800 Rockcreek Parkway Kansas City, MO 64117 816-201-1024 www.cerner.com	1997	Certified 7/18/06	Cerner Millennium - Fully integrated suite.	Anesthesiology, Endocrinology, Family Practice, Gastroenterology, Internal Medicine, Multi-Specialty.
PowerWorks Specialty	Cerner Corporation 2800 Rockcreek Parkway Kansas City, MO 64117 816-201-1024 www.cerner.com	1997		Cerner Practice Management.	Cardiology, Dermatology, Orthopaedics, Ophthalmology.
ChartLogic™ Electronic Medical Office	ChartLogic 3995 South 700 East, Suite 200 Salt Lake City , Utah 84107 801-365-1800/888-337-4441 www.chartlogic.com	2500 practices 1994		Many options	Orthopaedic, Optometric, 49 Specialty Specific Content
Essentris™ Acute Care	CliniComp International, Inc. 9655 Towne Centre Drive San Diego, CA 92121 800-350-8202 www.clinicomp.com	1983		HL7 supported hospital systems.	Hospitals
Touchscreen EHR - Electronic Health Record	ClinicPro Software 1438 N Hagadorn Rd. E Lansing, MI 48823 866-333-2776 www.clinicpro.com	30 Practices 1994		ClinicPro PMS	Chiropractic Software

Continued

EMR Product	Contact Information (Company, Address, Phone, Website)	Number of Installations/ Company Founded	CCHIT Status	PMS Options	Key Clinical Areas
MEDENT 17 EMR/EHR	Community Computer Service P.O. Box 980 Auburn, NY 13021 315-255-1751 www.medent.com	1,700 + 1968	Certified 7/31/06	MEDENT Practice Management	Medical content, for more than thirty different specialties
Eyecare Advantage, Ophthalmology Advantage	Compulink Business Systems, Inc. 2645 Townsgate Road, Suite 200 Westlake Village, CA 91361 800-456-4522 www.compulink-software.com	4,300 Practices 1985	In Process	Integrated with Compulink PMS.	Optometry, Ophthalmology, Physical Therapy, Podiatry, General Practitioner, University Healthcare Centers.
Medical Practice EMR 14	CPSI 6600 Wall St. Mobile, AL 36695 800-711-2774 www.cpsinet.com	1979	Certified 10/23/06		Hospitals
CureMD 9.0	CureMD Corporation 55 Broad Street New York, NY 10004 212- 509-6200 www.curemd.com	1997	Certified 4/30/2007	CureMD Practice Management System. HL7 interface for third party integration.	Allergy, Audiology, Cardiology, Dermatology, Emergency Medicine, Endocrinology, General Surgery, Hand Surgery, Infectious Disease, Internal Medicine, Neurology, Obstetrics/ Gynecology, Oncology, Ophthalmology, Orthopedics, Otolaryngology, Pain Management, Pediatrics, Physical Medicine, Podiatry, Primary Care, Family Practice, Rehabilitative Medicine, Rheumatology, Speech Therapy, Urology, Vascular Surgery, Nursing, Student and Employee Health Care Services, Sleep, Pulmonary

Continued

EMR Product	Contact Information (Company, Address, Phone, Website)	Number of Installations/ Company Founded	CCHIT Status	PMS Options	Key Clinical Areas
Dairyland's Clinical Information Management	Dairyland Healthcare Solutions 625 South Lakeshore Drive Glenwood, MN 56334 800-323-6987 www.dhsnet.com	400+ Hospitals 1980	In Process	Dairyland HIS	
ConnxtMD	DataHouse, Inc. 2001 Vendovi Lane Bellingham, WA 98229 888-327-2357 www.datahouse.com	1975		Misys PM, TeamPraxis, ConnxtMD. HL7 Integration	
Oacis EHR solution	DINMAR - (See Emergis)				
vxVisitA V1.0	Document Storage Systems, Inc. 12575 US Hwy 1, Suite 200 Juno Beach, FL 33408 561-227-0207 www.docstorsys.com	1996	Certified 4/30/07		Infectious Disease, Mental Health, Oncology, Pain Management, Anesthesia, Dental, Radiology.
eClinicalWorks Version 7.0 Release 2	eClinicalWorks Westborough Executive Park 112 Turnpike Road, Ste. 200 Westborough, MA 01581 508-836-2700/866-888-6929 www.eclinicalworks.com	3,000 1999	Certified 7/18/06	Integrated with eClinicalWorks, A4, SSIMED, Centricity, IDX.	Internists, Pediatricians, Family Practice, OB, and specialists.
eClinicalWorks Version 7.5	eClinicalWorks Westborough Executive Park 112 Turnpike Road, Ste. 200 Westborough, MA 01581 508-836-2700/866-888-6929 www.eclinicalworks.com	1999	Certified 2/6/07		
Sunrise Ambulatory Care 4.5	Eclipsys Corporation 1750 Clint Moore Road Boca Raton, FL 33487 561-322-4321 www.eclipsys.com	1,500+ Practices 1995	Certified 10/23/06	Sunrise™ Access Manager/Patient Financial Manager	Critical Care, Nursing, Radiology, Surgical.
CareRevolution 5.0i	EHS One Metroplex Dr., Ste. 500 Birmingham, Alabama 35209 205-871-1031/888-879-7302 www.ehsmed.com	350 Practices 1995	Certified 10/23/06	Integrated with Practice Revolution	Orthopedics, Cardiology, Podiatry.
e-MDs Solutions Series 6.1	e-MDs 500 West Whitestone Blvd. Cedar Park, TX 78613 888-344-9836/512-257-5200 www.e-mds.com	1996	Certified 7/18/06	Integrated with e-MDs Bill.	

Continued

EMR Product	Contact Information (Company, Address, Phone, Website)	Number of Installations/ Company Founded	CCHIT Status	PMS Options	Key Clinical Areas
MDAware® 2.2	eMedicalFiles, Inc. 7100 Peachtree Dunwoody Road, NE Atlanta, GA 30328 888-290-7565 www.emedicalfiles.com	2000	Certified 4/30/07	MDAware® practice management	
Oacis EMR	Emergis 1000, rue de Sérigny bureau 600 Longueuil, Quebec J4K 5B1 450-928-6000/866-363-7447 www.emergis.com	1992		Industry standard communications protocols are deployed such as HL7, CCOW, etc.	
TouchChart 3.3	Encite Johnstown, Pennsylvania 800-714-7199 www.encite.us	2004	Certified 1/29/07		
EpicCare Ambulatory EMR Spring 2006	Epic Systems Corporation 5301 Tokay Blvd. Madison, WI 53711-1027 608-271-9000 www.epicsystems.com	150+ groups 1979	Certified 7/18/06	Resolute Professional Billing, Cadense. Also interfaces with other products	Emergency Medicine, Cardiology, others.
MaximEyes EMR	First Insight Corp. 22845 NW Bennett St. Suite 200, Building B Hillsboro, OR 97124 800-920-1940 www.first-insight.com	4,500 + Providers 1994		MaximEyes PMS	Optometrists, Ophthalmologists and Opticians.
MediNotes e Electronic Medical Records	Fox Meadows Software 400 Arbor Lake Dr., Suite B600 Columbia, SC 29223 877-369-3282/803-736-8000 www.foxmeadows.com	4300 1994	Accepted Oct. 2006	Encounter Manager, MediSoft, Centricity, Lytec, Medical Manager, and more.	Cardiology, Chiropractic, Dermatology, Family Medicine, Internal Medicine, Neurology, OG-GYN, Ophthalmology, Optometry, Orthopedics, Otolaryngology, Pediatrics, Podiatry, Primary Care, Rheumatology, Surgery and Urology.
Centricity® EMR 2005 Version 6.0	GE Medical Systems 8200 W. Tower Ave. Milwaukee, WI 53223 414-355-5000 www.gemedical.com	750+ practices	Certified 7/18/06	Partner with Centricity PMS (formerly Millbrook)	Links with other PMS products.

Continued

EMR Product	Contact Information (Company, Address, Phone, Website)	Number of Installations/ Company Founded	CCHIT Status	PMS Options	Key Clinical Areas
Centricity® Practice Solution Version 6.0	GE Medical Systems 8200 W. Tower Ave. Milwaukee, WI 53223 414-355-5000 www.gemedical.com		Certified 3/28/07		
GlaceEMR 2.0	Glenwood Systems, LLC 81 West Main St., W Wing 3rd Fl. Waterbury CT 06702 888-Glace-MD www.glaceemr.com	1998	Certified 4/30/07		Internal Medicine, Pediatrics, OB/GYN, Cardiology, Neurology, Nephrology, Psychiatry, Pulmonology, Pain Management, General Surgery, Orthopedics, Urology, ENT.
gloEMR 3.5	gloStream, Inc. 6632 Telegraph Road Suite 363 Bloomfield Hills, MI 48301 877-gloEMR1 www.glostream.com		Certified 4/30/07	Standards-based HL7 protocol.	Cardiology Orthopedics Sports medicine Family practice OB/GYN Neurology Urology ENT Gastroenterology Dermatology Hematology Rheumatology Plastic Surgery Internal Medicine Pediatrics
PrimeSuite® 2007	Greenway Medical Technologies 121 Greenway Blvd. Carrollton, GA 30117 770-836-3100 www.greenwaymedical.com	215+ practices 1998	Certified 10/23/07	Integrated with PrimeSuite/PrimePractice.	OBGYN, Prenatal, Urology, General Surgery, and General/Family Practices.
mMD.Net EHR 9.0.9	Health Communication Systems, LLC Corporate Office 11 Compton Court, Suite 200 Perrineville, NJ 08535 800-741-0981 www.healthcomsys.com		Certified 7/18/06	Integrates with existing applications and utilizes hardware and networks already deployed through state-of-the-art middleware and Internet technologies.	

Continued

EMR Product	Contact Information (Company, Address, Phone, Website)	Number of Installations/ Company Founded	CCHIT Status	PMS Options	Key Clinical Areas
HealthPort EHR v8.5 (formerly Companion EMR v8.5)	HealthPort P.O Box 100114 Columbia, SC 29202 800 999-0788 x1173 www.healthport.com		Certified 7/18/06	HealthPort PM	Health Centers, Orthopedics, Other Specialty Specific Content
MicroMD EMR 5.0	Henry Schein Medical Systems 760 Boardman-Canfield Rd. Boardman, OH 44512 800.624.8832 www.micromd.com	1982	Certified 1/29/07	MicroMD®	
iMedica Patient Relationship Manager 2006, version 6.0	iMedica 4699 Old Ironsides Dr. Suite 450 Santa Clara, CA 95054 866-960-6890 www.imedica.com	50 Practices 1998	Certified 11/15/06	Interfaces with other Practice Management Systems thru HL7.	Primary Care and Specialties.
Multi-ACCESS™	IMPAC Medical Systems, Inc. 100 West Evelyn Avenue Mountain View, CA 94041 800-488-4672 www.impac.com	800+ Practices 1990		Integrated PMS and EMR. Interfaces with other products through HL7.	Oncology, Radiology, Pathology, Lab.
Praxis Electronic Medical Records, version 3.5	Infor-Med Medical Information Systems Warner Center 6271 Variel Avenue, Suite A Woodland Hills, CA 91367-2512 800-985-6016 www.praxisemr.com	3300 Practices 1989	Certified 7/31/06	ASTM section 14.01 and HL7 standards. Integrates with most Practice Management Systems.	Nephrology, Urology, Family Practice, Pain Management, General Surgery.
Physicians' Workstation Suite (PWS)	Integrated Healthware, LLC 101 Billerica Avenue, Building 5 North Billerica, MA 01862-1271 888-813-7575 www.ihealthware.com	200+ Practices 1997		Partner with Entity PMS. Interfaced with other PMS products thru HL7 exchanges.	Several Specialties
OmniMD EMR 6.0.5	Integrated Systems Management, Inc. 303 South Broadway, Suite 101 Tarrytown, NY 10591 914-332-5590 www.omnimd.com	300 practices 1989	Certified 4/30/07	Integrates with other PMS products thru HL7.	Cardiology, Dermatology, Endocrinology, Gastroenter-ology, Family Practice, Internal Medicine, Neur-ology, OB/GYN, Ophthalmology, Orthopedics, Pain Manage-ment, Pediatrics, Psychiatry, Pulm-onology, Urology.

Continued

EMR Product	Contact Information (Company, Address, Phone, Website)	Number of Installations/ Company Founded	CCHIT Status	PMS Options	Key Clinical Areas
IC-Chart Release 6.0	InteGreat, Inc. 14988 North 78th Way, #100 Scottsdale, AZ 85260-3476 800-676-1360 www.igreat.com	15 Clinics 1998	Certified 1/29/07	Links thru HL7 and proprietary interfaces.	Multi Specialty, Radiology.
OfficeEMR 2007	iSALUS Healthcare 212 West 10th Street Suite B120 Indianapolis, IN 46202 888-280-6678 iSALUShealthcare.com	2000	Certified 4/30/07	ASP Full Service Solution.	
EncounterPRO EHR 5.0	JMJ Technologies, Inc. 2000 RiverEdge Parkway Suite GL 100A Atlanta, GA 30328 770-919-7220/800-677-5653 www.jmjtech.com	270 Practices 1994	Certified 7/18/06	Workflow Management System (WfMS). Navigational (More intuitive than MDI).	Allergy and Immunology, Family Medicine, Internal Medicine, Obstetrics and Gynecology, Pediatrics, Ophthalmology, Neurology.
KeyChart®	KeyMedical Software, Inc. 1700 North Lebanon St. P.O. Box 588 Lebanon, IN 46052 765-482-7964/888-953-9633 www.keymedicalsoftware.net	1987		KeyMed, eCeno (MedEvolve), PRISM, Medical Manager, Cro-well. Interface using HL7 data exchange stan-dards.	Ophthalmology
LifeT.I.M.E. (7.100)	LifeWatch Technologies, Inc. - A LifeWatch Corp Company 1351A Abbott Court Buffalo Grove, IL 60089 (877) 774-9846 www.lifewatchinc.com	1983	Certified 1/29/07		

Continued

EMR Product	Contact Information (Company, Address, Phone, Website)	Number of Installations/ Company Founded	CCHIT Status	PMS Options	Key Clinical Areas
LifeT.I.M.E. (7.100)	LifeWatch Technologies, Inc. - A LifeWatch Corp Company 1351A Abbott Court Buffalo Grove, IL 60089 (877) 774-9846 www.lifewatchinc.com	1983	Certified 1/29/07		
Medical and Practice Management (MPM) Suite MAGIC Version 5.5	LSS Data Systems 6423 City West Parkway Eden Prairie, MN 55344-3246 952-941-1000 www.lssdata.com	1982	Certified 1/29/2007	MEDITECH's HCIS - Meditech and LSS Medical and Practice Management (MPM) Suite	
CattailsMD Version 5	Marshfield Clinic 1000 North Oak Avenue Marshfield, WI 54449 800-782-8581 x1-8164 www.cattailsmd.com www.marshfieldclinic.org		Certified 1/29/07		
Horizon Ambulatory Care™ Version 9.4	McKesson Provider Technologies 5995 Windward Parkway Alpharetta, GA 30005 404.338.6000 www.mckesson.com		Certified 7/18/06	McKesson's Horizon Practice Solutions Suite	
MDLAND Electronic Health Record and Practice Management Systems 8.0	MDLAND 40 Exchange Place 8th Floor New York, NY 10005 212-684-9038 www.mdland.com	1999	Certified 4/30/07		
MD Logic	MD Logic, Inc. 2170 Satellite Blvd., Suite 435 Duluth, GA 30097 800-273-7750/770-497-1560 www.mdlogic.com	1,400 Practices 1994		Interfaced with several PMS products through HL7 exchanges.	General Surgery Hand Surgery Hematology Infectious Disease Internal Medicine Multi-Specialty Groups Neurology Neurosurgery OB-GYN Oncology Cardiology Endocrinology ENT Otolaryngology Family Practice Ophthalmology Optometry

Continued

EMR Product	Contact Information (Company, Address, Phone, Website)	Number of Installations/ Company Founded	CCHIT Status	PMS Options	Key Clinical Areas
					Orthopaedic Otology Pain Management Pediatrics Physiatry Physical Therapy Plastic Surgery Podiatry Primary Care Radiation Oncology Spine Urology Vascular
MDTABLET 2.6.7	MDTablet 1836 Lackland Hill Parkway St. Louis, MO 63146 888-989-1965 www.mdtablet.com	1991	Certified 4/30/07		
MEDAZ 60720.001	MedAZ.Net, LLC (wholly owned subsidiary of Koni Ameri Tech Services, Inc) 37 Station Drive, Suite 1E Princeton Junction, NJ 08550 888-633 2972 www.MedAZ.net		Certified 1/29/07	MedAZ Practice Management Suite	
Welford Chart Notes	MEDCOM Information Systems, Inc. 2117 Stonington Avenue. Hoffman Estates, IL 60195 800-213-2161 www.emirj.com	200+ Practices 1991		Partner with Edimis Practice Manager Interfaced with other PMSs through HL7 exchanges.	Primary Care
MedcomSoft® Record 2006™	MedcomSoft Inc. 5355 Hunter Road Atlanta, GA 30349 877-673-0101 www.medcomsoft.com	1994	Certified 7/18/06	Includes integrated PMS system. Also interfaces with: IDX, KMS, Lytec, MD Office, Medical Manager, MediSoft, Medstar, Millbrook.	26 Specialty Modules, incl. Allergy and Rheumatology, Orthopaedics, Cardiology, Dermatology, Pediatrics, Gastroenterology, Physical Therapy, Neurology, Radiology, OB/GYN, Oncology, Urology, Ophthalmology

Continued

EMR Product	Contact Information (Company, Address, Phone, Website)	Number of Installations/ Company Founded	CCHIT Status	PMS Options	Key Clinical Areas
WebChart 4.23	Medical Informatics Engineering 6302 Constitution Drive Fort Wayne, Indiana 46804 260-459-6270 www.mieweb.com	1995	Certified 7/18/06		
Medical Messenger Astral Jet EMR 3.7.1	Medical Messenger 800-965-9959 Web site under re-design		Certified 4/30/07		
harmony e/Notes (EMR)	Medical Technology International 800-777-7684 www.medtec.net				23 Specialty Modules
Medicat 8.8	Medicat 1100 Johnson Ferry Rd. Suite. 240 Atlanta, GA 30342 866- 633-4053 www.medicat.com	1993	Certified 1/29/07		College Health
MedicWare EMR 7	MedicWare, Inc 6520 North Irwindale Ave. Suite 215 Irwindale, CA 91702 626-334-5678 www.medicware.com	100+ Practices 1991	Certified 1/29/07	Interfaces with other PMS products through HL7 exchanges.	Internal Medicine, Urology, Pediatrics, Orthopaedics, and others.
MedInformatix V 6.0	MedInformatix, Inc 5777 W. Century Blvd, Suite 1700 Los Angeles, CA 90045 310-348-7367 www.medinformatix.com	800+ Practices 1992	Certified 1/29/07	Integrated with MedInformatix PMS.	Ophthalmology, Pediatrics, Radiology, Cardiology, Internal Medicine.
MediNotes e 5.0	MediNotes Corporation 1025 Ashworth Road, Suite 222 West Des Moines, IA 50265 877-633-6683 www.medinotes.com	4,000 Practices 1997	Certified 10/23/06	Interfaces with other products via HL7 ex-changes.	Most Specialties, OB/GYN, Neurology, Orthopaedics, Ophthalmology, Opticians, Pediatrics.
Intelligent Medical Software (IMS) 2007	Meditab Software, Inc. 333 Hegenberger Road, Suite 800 Oakland, CA 94621 510-632-8021/866-994-6367 www.meditab.com	1998	Certified 1/29/07	Fully integrated EMR and Prac-tice Manage-ment software for single and multi- physician facilities.	Allergy, Cardi-ology, Diabetes, Endocrinology, Family Practice, Internal Medi-cine, Oncology, Ophthalmology, Pain, Pediatric, Psychiatry

Continued

EMR Product	Contact Information (Company, Address, Phone, Website)	Number of Installations/ Company Founded	CCHIT Status	PMS Options	Key Clinical Areas
MedPlexus EHR 8.5	MedPlexus, Inc. 1263 Oakmead Parkway Sunnyvale, CA 95085 408-990-9080 www.medplexus.com	50+ Practices 2000	Certified 10/23/06	Interfaced with MedPlexus Practice Management System and third-party practice management systems.	Family Practice and Internal Medicine, Cardiology, OB/GYN, Women's Health, Neurology, Pediatrics, Gastroenterology.
EMRWorks Electronic Medical Record (EMR)	MedStar Systems 3115 NW 10th Terrace Suite 104 Fort Lauderdale, FL 33309 866-775-7779/954-332-0520 www.medstarsystems.com	66 Practices		Integrated with MedStar PMS. Interfaced with other PMS products thru HL7 exchanges.	Surgery, Orthopaedic, ENT.
meridianEMR 3.6.1	meridianEMR, Inc. 354 Eisenhower Parkway Livingston, NJ 07039 877 411-4367 www.meridianEMR.com		Certified 4/30/07	Integrated with meridianPractice Management System. Interface with any commercially viable HL7 compliant PM system.	Urology, General Surgery, Internal Medicine
Misys EMR 8.0	Misys Healthcare Systems 8529 Six Forks Road Raleigh, NC 27615 866-647-9787 www.misyshealthcare.com	400 Practices 1979	Certified 7/18/06	Partner product to MISYS PMS.	Variety of specialties and primary care.
dChart EMR 4.5	NCG Medical Systems, Inc. 140 North Westmonte Dr. Altamonte Springs, FL 32714 800-959-1906 www.ncgmedical.com	1999	Certified 2/9/07	Optional complete Work Flow module and has a back-office component. Interfaces with Perfect Care, Medical Manager, Mysis, Medisoft, Lytec, Medmaster, CDL, MOS, and others.	
NextGen EMR 5.3	NextGen Healthcare Info. Sys. 795 Horsham Rd., 2nd Floor Horsham, PA 19044 215-657-7010 www.nextgen.com	1200 Practices	Certified 7/18/06	Integrated with Enterprise Practice Management (EPM). Interfaces with other PMS products through HL7 exchanges.	Variety of specialties and primary care.

Continued

EMR Product	Contact Information (Company, Address, Phone, Website)	Number of Installations/ Company Founded	CCHIT Status	PMS Options	Key Clinical Areas
Nightingale PWS (formerly *Physicians' Workstation Suite*)	Nightingale Informatix Corporation 3760 14th Avenue, Suite 200 Markham, Ontario L3R 3T7 905-943-2600/866-852-3663 www.nightingale.md	2002	Certified 7/18/06	Offers a fully integrated Internet-based Electronic Health Record (EHR), Electronic Medical Record (EMR) and Practice Management solution. Interfaces to Ridge-Mark and Entity Practice Management applications.	
Noteworthy EHR 5.4	Noteworthy Medical Systems, Inc. 6001 Landerhaven Dr., Unit D Cleveland, OH 44124 800-224-9740/440-684-6800 www.noteworthyehr.com	1997	Certified 10/23/06	Interfaces seamlessly with any practice management system and numerous hospital applications, databases and external systems through Orion Health's Rhapsody interface engine.	
Longitudinal Medical Record (LMR) 5.1.1	Partners HealthCare System, Inc. 978-741-1200	1994			
EpiChart 5.2	Polaris Medical Management, Inc. 180 Norwood Ave. Cranston, RI 02905 401-781-7810 www.PolarisMedical.com	1998	Certified 4/30/07	Interface via HL7, ANSI.	
PowerMed EMR	PowerMed Corp. 48 Free Street Portland, Maine 04101 207-772-3920/888-621-5565 www.powermed.com	1990's	Certified 4/30/07	PowerMed - Fully integrated suite. Mac and Windows based.	Allergy & Immunization, Cardiology, Ob-Gyn, Orthopaedics, Ophthalmology.
e-Medsys EHR	Practice One 21515 Vanowen Street Suite 250 Canoga Park, CA 91303 www.practiceone.com	250 Practices	Certified 2007	E-Medsys PMS	Cardiology Family Practice Gastroenterology Internal Medicine Oncology Urology

Continued

EMR Product	Contact Information (Company, Address, Phone, Website)	Number of Installations/ Company Founded	CCHIT Status	PMS Options	Key Clinical Areas
Practice Partner Patient Records	Practice Partner (Formerly Physician Micro Systems) 2401 4th Avenue, Suite 700 Seattle, WA 98121 800-770-7674/206-441-2400 www.practicepartner.com	1,500 Practices 1983	Certified 7/18/06	Practice Partner /Total Practice. Also interfaces with other PMS products via HL7.	Primary Care
Patient Chart Manager	Prime Clinical Systems, Inc. 3675 E. Huntington Drive, Suite A Pasadena, CA 91107 800-523-5977/626-449-1705 www.primeclinical.com	600 Practices 1983	Certified 4/30/07	OnStaff PMS	Supports most specialties.
StreamlineMD™ ProPractica, Inc.	20600 Chagrin Blvd. Suite 400 Shaker Heights, OH 44122 216-373-7390 www.propractica.com		Certified 10/23/06		
Pulse Patient Relationship Management (Pulse PRM)	Pulse Systems, Inc. 3017 North Cypress Wichita, KS 67226 800-444-0882 www.pulseinc.com	290 Practices 1982	Certified 1/29/07	Pulse PRM is a fully Integrated suite. Also interfaces with other PMS products via HL7.	
MediTalk Enterprise	Quincy Systems 1502 East 17th Street Suite B Georgetown, TX 78626 888-346-6842 www.quincysys.com	247 Sites/530 Providers 1997	Will apply in 2008.	Have written interfaces for most PMS products.	32 Specialties including Orthopaedic Surgery, Cardiology, Pain Management.
Intergy EHR by Sage	Sage Software Healthcare, Inc. 2202 N. West Shore Blvd. Suite 300 Tampa, FL 33607-5749 877-932-6301 www.sagehealth.com	1982	Certified 7/18/06	Interfaces with other PMS products via HL7.	Cardiology, Gastroenterology, GYN, Nephrology, Neurology, Orthopaedics, Radiology, Urology.
SequelMed EMR V7.50	Sequel Systems, Inc. 225 BroadHollow Rd. Ste. 205E Melville, NY 11747 800-965-2728 www.sequelsys.com	1995	Certified 4/30/07	SequelMed EPM and ASP.	
SOAPware® The Electronic Health Record	SOAPware, Inc. 4220 N. Crossover Rd. Fayetteville, AR 72703 800-455-7627 http://docs.com	9,000+ 1995	Registering New Version in 2007	Lytec, Medisoft, SOAPware Scheduling. DOCSExchange, X-link.	

Continued

EMR Product	Contact Information (Company, Address, Phone, Website)	Number of Installations/ Company Founded	CCHIT Status	PMS Options	Key Clinical Areas
Emrge 6.0 Release 1.0	SSIMED, LLC 835 Bloomfield Avenue Windsor, CT 06095 860-688-0033 www.ssimed.com	1991	Certified 1/29/07	SSIMED Practice Manager™ suite. Interface via HL-7, ANSI, NSF.	Anesthesiology Radiology
ChartMaker®	STI Computer Services Inc. 2550 Eisenhower Ave. Bldg. C Norristown, PA 19403 610-650-9700 www.sticomputer.com	200 + Practices Serves Mid Atlantic Region. 1979	In Process	Perfect Care® for Windows Practice Management and Electronic Billing	Templates available for most specialties.
SRS Freedom Chart Manager	SRS Software, Inc. 180 Summit Avenue, Suite 203 Montvale, NJ 07645 201-802-1300 /800-288-8369 www.srssoft.com	250 Practices 1997		All major practice management software systems including A4 Health Systems, GE Centricity, IDX, Misys, Medical Manager, NextGen and WebMD, through HL7 exchanges.	Allergy and Rheumatology, Orthopaedics, Cardiology, Otolaryngology, Dermatology, Pediatrics, Gastroenterology, Physical Therapy, Neurology, Radiology, OB/GYN, Oncology, Urology, Ophthalmology, Optometry.
OrthoPad® Digital Patient Charts	Stryker Orthopaedics 325 Corporate Drive Mahwah, NJ 07430 201-831-5000 www.stryker.com/orthopaedics	325		Integration with DICOM and HL7 standards.	Orthopaedic Group Practices
SynaMed EMR	SynaMed 363 7th Ave. New York , NY 10001 866-SYNAMED/866-796-2633 www.synamed.com	300 + Practices	Certified 4/30/07	Web-based - Integrated with SynaMed PMS. Interfaces with other PMS products through HL7 exchanges.	
Clinician's Desktop™	The Echo Group PO Box 2150 15 Washington Street Conway, NH 03818 800-635-8209/603-447-8600 www.echoman.com	1980			Behavioral Healthcare Organizations

Continued

EMR Product	Contact Information (Company, Address, Phone, Website)	Number of Installations/ Company Founded	CCHIT Status	PMS Options	Key Clinical Areas
VersaSuite	Universal Software Solutions, Inc. VersaSuite US 13401 Pond Spring Road Austin, TX 78729 866-395-8774 www.versasuite.com	100 + 1994	Certified 1/29/07	VersaSuite PM VersaSuite Optical Interfaces with other PMS products via HL7.	Retail Optical
Pro-Filer 2007	UNI/CARE Systems, Inc. 540 North Tamiami Trail Sarasota, Florida 34236 941-954-3403 www.unicaresys.com	1981	Certified 4/30/07		Public Health, Foster/Residential Health, Adoption, Juvenile Justice, Behavioral Health, Mental Health, Substance Abuse, Developmental Disabilities, Mental Retardation, Primary Care, Disease Management, Rehabilitation,
Endosoft	Utech Products, Inc. EndoSoft (A Division of Utech Products, Inc.) 135 Broadway Schenectady NY 12305 518-831-8000 www.endosoft.com		Certified 4/30/07	EndoSoft OBPM suite. HL7, DICOM, VISTA interfaces.	Gastroenterology, Pulmonary, Orthopedics, Pain Management, Podiatry, Plastic Surgery, General Surgery,ENT, Ophthalmology, Oral Surgery, Urology, OB/GYN, Cardiology, Dermatology, Wound Management, Pathology.
ChartKeeper	VantageMed Corporation 3017 Kilgore Rd., Suite 180 Rancho Cordova, CA 95670 800-343-5737/877-879-8633 724-935-5000-Anesthesia products www.vantagemed.com	1,200 Practices 2002		Interfaces with other PMS products via HL7.	Anesthesiology, Behavioral Health
Visionary Dream EHR 7.1	Visionary Medical Systems, Inc. 5600 Mariner St, Suite 227 Tampa, FL 33609 813-594-1026/888-895-2466 www.visionarymed.com	200 Practices 1996	Certified 1/29/2007	Interfaced with Visionary Office PM.	Primary Care

Continued

EMR Product	Contact Information (Company, Address, Phone, Website)	Number of Installations/ Company Founded	CCHIT Status	PMS Options	Key Clinical Areas
Waiting Room Solutions EMR	Waiting Room Solutions 1 Harriman Dr Medical Arts Building #1 Goshen, NY 10924 866-977-4367 www.waitingroomsolutions.com		Certified 4/30/07	Waiting Room Solutions Practice Management System is a web-based PMS & EMR solution.	ENT, Allergy, Audiology.
WEBeDoctor® Physician-office®	WEBeDoctor 471 West Lambert Road, Ste. 102 Brea, CA 92821 714-990-3999 www.webedoctor.com	1999			
workflow EHR	Workflow.com, LLC 24651 Center Ridge Road, Suite 575 Westlake, Ohio 44145 877-438-9332/440-808-2700 www.workflow.com	2002	Certified 4/30/07	Workflow PM HL7 interface.	
WorldVistA EHR™	WorldVistA - (System was originally developed by the U.S. Department of Veterans Affairs (VA)) P.O. Box 131912 Houston, Texas 77219 www.worldvista.org	2002	Certified 4/30/07		Pediatrics, OB/GYN.

GLOSSARY

Cluster Server—A cluster server is actually two separate computers that maintain the EMR. One of the servers is the active server and the second mimics the first server. If the primary server fails, the second server becomes the primary server.

Hot Swap Disk Drive—Hot swap disks offer a fail-safe option for EMRs. Hot swap disks are typically used in redundant disk setups. Pairs of hot swap disks are used to store the same information. If one of the disks fails, you can remove it and replace it with a new disk. The system will automatically copy the contents of the working disk to the new disk.

Go Live—The point when your practice is using the EMR as the primary repository of clinical information in the practice.

PMS—Practice Management Systems (PMS) typically includes an appointment scheduler and allows for processing of charges and payments.